Case Studies in Reproduction

Common and Uncommon Presentations

Case Studies in Assisted Reproduction

Common and Uncommon Presentations

Nick S. Macklon
University of Southampton, UK

Human M. Fatemi
The Centre for Reproductive Medicine, NOVA-IVI Fertility, Abu Dhabi/UAE

Robert J. Norman
The University of Adelaide, Australia

Pasquale Patrizio
Yale School of Medicine, New Haven, CT, USA

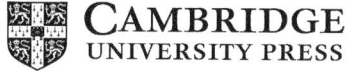

CAMBRIDGE
UNIVERSITY PRESS

University Printing House, Cambridge CB2 8BS, United Kingdom

Cambridge University Press is part of the University of Cambridge.

It furthers the University's mission by disseminating knowledge in the pursuit of education, learning and research at the highest international levels of excellence.

www.cambridge.org
Information on this title: www.cambridge.org/9781107664579

First published 2015

A catalogue record for this publication is available from the British Library

Library of Congress Cataloguing in Publication data
Case studies in assisted reproduction : common and uncommon presentations / [edited by] Nick S. Macklon, Human M. Fatemi, Robert J. Norman, Pasquale Patrizio.
    p. ; cm.
Includes bibliographical references and index.
ISBN 978-1-107-66457-9 (paperback)
I. Macklon, Nick S., editor.   II. Fatemi, Human M., editor.   III. Norman, Robert (Robert J.), editor.   IV. Patrizio, Pasquale., editor.
[DNLM: 1. Reproductive Techniques, Assisted–Case Reports.   2. Genital Diseases, Female–complications–Case Reports.   3. Genital Diseases, Male–complications–Case Reports.   4. Infertility–Case Reports. WQ 208]
RG133.5
618.1'78–dc23
2014036818

ISBN 978-1-107-66457-9 Paperback

....

Contents

Contributors

Masoud Azodi
Department of OB/GYN and Reproductive Sciences, Gynecologic Oncology Section, Yale University School of Medicine, New Haven, CT, USA

Patricia Baetens
Psychologist at the Centre for Reproductive Medicine at the Universitair Ziekenhuis Brussel (UZ Brussel) Brussels, Belgium

Steven Bayer
Boston IVF Inc., Waltham, MA, USA

Joel Bernstein
Medical Director at Fertility East, Sydney, NSW, Australia

Jonathan D. Black
Physician, Department of Obstetrics, Gynecology, and Reproductive Sciences, Yale University School of Medicine, New Haven, CT, USA

Christophe Blockeel
Medical director/gynecologist at the Centre for Reproductive Medicine at Universitair Ziekenhuis Brussel (UZ Brussel), Brussels, Belgium

Carolien M. Boomsma
Specialist training fellow in Obstetrics and Gynecology, University Medical Center Utrecht, The Netherlands

Birgit Borgström
Department of Pediatrics, Karolinska Institute, Stockholm, Sweden

Mark Bowman
Fertility Specialist, Genea, NSW, Australia

Nicholas Brook
Complete Fertility Centre, University Hospitals Southampton NHS Foundation Trust, Southampton, UK

Elisabeth Carlsen
The Fertility Clinic, Copenhagen University Hospital, Denmark

Peter Carne
Colorectal Surgeon, Cabrini and Alfred Hospitals; Senior Lecturer, Cabrini Monash University Department of Surgery, VIC, Australia

Ying Cheong
Associate Professor of Obstetrics and Gynaecology, University of Southampton, and Clinical Director, Complete Fertility Centre, Southampton, UK

Jen-Ruei Chen
Division of Gynecologic Oncology, Department of OB/GYN, Mackay Memorial Hospital, Taipei, and Mackay Medicine, Nursing and Management College, Taipei, Taiwan, ROC

Erin Clark
Consultant Physician in Obstetric Medicine, Women's and Children's Hospital, Adelaide, SA, Australia

S. Alberto Dávila Garza
Instituto para el Estudio de la Concepción Humana, IECH, Monterrey, Mexico

Sunita De Sousa
Endocrine Fellow, University of Adelaide School of Medicine, Adelaide, SA, South Australia

Michel De Vos
Medical director/gynecologist at the Center for Reproductive Medicine, Universitair Ziekenhuis Brussel (UZ Brussel), Brussels, Belgium

Leo Doherty
IVF New Jersey, Somerset, NJ, USA

Patricio Donoso
Reproductive Medicine Unit, Clinica Alemana, Vitacura 5951, Santiago, Chile

Cindy M. P. Duke
Clinical Instructor, Reproductive Endocrinology & Infertility, Department. of Obstetrics and Gynecology, Yale University School of Medicine, New Haven, CT, USA

Human M. Fatemi
Professor of Reproductive Medicine at the Centre for Reproductive Medicine, NOVA-IVI Fertility, Abu Dhabi/UAE

Alison Fernbach
Pediatric Nurse Practitioner, Division of Pediatric Hematology/Oncology/Stem cell transplantation, Morgan Stanley Children's Hospital of New York-Presbyterian, Columbia University Medical Center, NY, USA

Juan A. Garcia-Velasco
Professor of Obstetrics and Gynecology, IVI-Madrid, Rey Juan Carlos University, Madrid, Spain

Elizabeth S. Ginsburg
Medical Director of the In Vitro Fertilization Program at Brigham & Women's Hospital, and an Associate Professor of Obstetrics, Gynecology and Reproductive Biology at Harvard Medical School, MA, USA

Dorothy A. Greenfeld
Department of Obstetrics, Gynecology and Reproductive Science, Yale University School of Medicine, New Haven, CT, USA

William M. Hague
Professor – Robinson Research Institute; Professor of Obstetric Medicine, School of Paediatrics and Reproductive Health, University of Adelaide; Senior Consultant Physician in Obstetric Medicine, Women & Children's Hospital, Adelaide, SA, Australia

Daniel Hajioff
North Bristol NHS Trust, Bristol, UK

Tristan Hardy
Obstetric and Gynecology fellow, Royal Hospital for Women, University of New South Wales, Sydney, Australia

Catherine Henry
Trainee in Internal Medicine, Royal Adelaide Hospital, Adelaide, SA, Australia

Outi Hovatta
Senior professor of Obstetrics, Department of Obstetrics and Gynecology, Karolinska Institute, Stockholm, Sweden

John Hutton
Professor of Reproductive Endocrinology and Infertility, University of Otago, Wellington, New Zealand

Gordana Ivanovic
Special Gynecological Hospital 'Ivanovic' Belgrade, Serbia

Sameer Jatkar
Fellow in Reproductive Medicine, Monash IVF, Richmond, VIC, Australia

Shilpa Jesudason
Consultant physician, Renal Medicine, Central and Northern Adelaide Renal and Transplantation Service, The Royal Adelaide Hospital, Adelaide, SA, Australia

Theo Joseph
Royal National Throat, Nose and Ear Hospital, London, UK

Amanda Kallen
Assistant Professor, Obstetrics, Gynecology, and Reproductive Sciences at the Department of Obstetrics, Gynecology & Reproductive Sciences, Yale School of Medicine, New Haven, CT, USA

Sonal Karia
Fertility Specialist, Genea, NSW, Australia

Bala Karunakaran
University Hospitals Southampton NHS Foundation Trust, Southampton,UK

Jenneke C. Kasius
Department of Reproductive Medicine and Gynecology, University Medical Center Utrecht, Utrecht, The Netherlands.

Ben Kroon
Queensland Fertility Group Research Foundation and the University of Queensland, Queensland, Australia

Dimitra Kyrou
Specialist in Reproductive Medicine, Clinical Director of Assisted Reproduction Unit 'Assisting Nature', Thessaloniki, Greece

Robert Lahoud
Clinical Director, IVFAustralia, Castle Hill, NSW, Australia

Jennifer M Levine
Medical Director, Center for Survivor Wellness, Assistant Professor of Pediatrics at Columbia University Medical Center Division of Hematology, Oncology and Stem Cell Transplant

Inge Liebaers
Emeritus professor in medical genetics, former Director of the Center for Medical Genetics, Vrije Universiteit Brussels, Brussels, Belgium

Shane T. Lipskind
Arizona Center for Fertility Studies, Scottsdale, Arizona, USA

Derek Lok
Fertility Specialist, Genea, NSW, Australia

Nick S. Macklon
Professor of Obstetrics and Gynaecology, University of Southampton, UK

Manveen (Manny) Mangat
Specialist in Infertility & IVF, Laparoscopic Surgery, Male Infertility and Gynecology, North Shore Specialist Day Hospital, North Shore Private and Mater Private, and IVFAustralia's City and Northshore clinics, Sydney, NSW, Australia

Tom P. Manolitsas
Gynecologist, Epworth Eastern Hospital, Box Hill, VIC, Australia

S. McDowell
Queensland Fertility Group Research Foundation and University of Queensland, Queensland, Australia

Cherise Mooy
Senior embryologist, IVFAustralia, Sydney, NSW, Australia

Mark R. Morton
Senior consultant physician in Obstetric Medicine, Women's and Children's Hospital, North Adelaide, SA, Australia

Andrew Murray
Medial Director, Fertility Associates, Wellington; Senior Lecturer, Otago School of Medicine, Wellington, New Zealand

Robert J. Norman
Professor of Reproductive and Periconceptual Medicine, Robinson Research Institute, Department of Obstetrics & Gynecology, University of Adelaide, SA, Australia

Sara Ornaghi
Department of Obstetrics and Gynecology, University of Milna-Bicocca and San Gerardo Hospital, Monza, Italy

Israel Ortega
IVI-Madrid, Rey Juan Carlos University, Madrid, Spain

Michael J. Paidas
Professor of Obstetrics, Gynecology, and Reproductive Sciences, Co-Director, Yale Women and Children's Center for Blood Disorders and Co-Director at the National Hemophilia Foundation-Baxter Clinical Fellowship at Yale School of Medicine, New Haven, CT, USA

Evaggelos Papanikolaou
Director, Human Reproduction and Genetics Foundation, Thessaloniki, Greece

Pasquale Patrizio
Professor of Obstetrics and Gynecology and Director, Yale Fertility Center, Yale University School of Medicine, New Haven, CT, USA

Sofie Piessens
Camberwell Ultrasound for Women, Hawthorn East, and Central Ultrasound for Women, Fitzroy, VIC, Australia

Biljana Popovic Todorovic
Fertility specialist at IVF Center "Ivanovic", Belgrade, Serbia

Luk Rombauts
Adjunct Clinical Associate Professor in the Department of Obstetrics and Gynecology at Monash University and the Head of Reproductive Medicine at Monash Medical Centre, Southern Health, Melbourne, VIC, Australia

Katrina Rowan
Fertility specialist, Genea, NSW, Australia

Denny Sakkas
Boston IVF Inc., Waltham, MA, USA

P. Sanhueza
Reproductive Medicine Unit, Clinica Alemana, Vitacura 5951, Santiago, Chile

Kirsten Tryde Schmidt
Consultant Gynecologist, Fertility Clinic, University Hospital of Copenhagen (Rigshospitalet), Copenhagen, Denmark

Mark Teoh
Camberwell Ultrasound for Women, Hawthorn East, and Central Ultrasound for Women, Fitzroy, VIC, Australia

Hammed A. Tijani
Senior Special Interest Training Fellow, Obstetrics and Gynecology Department, University Hospitals Southampton NHS, Southampton, UK.

Jelena Todorovic
Fertility specialist at IVF Center "Ivanovic", Belgrade, Serbia

Saioa Torrealday
Clinical Instructor, Department of Obstetrics, Gynecology and Reproductive Science, Yale University School of Medicine, New Haven, CT, USA

Herman Tournaye
Professor in Reproductive Medicine, Developmental Biology and Embryology at Vrije Universiteit Brussel and Director of the Center for Reproductive Medicine at Universitair Ziekenhuis Brussel (UZ Brussel), Brussels, Belgium

Geoffrey Trew
Institute of Reproductive and Developmental Biology, Hammersmith Hospital, London, UK

W. Verpoest
Medical Director/gynaecologist at the Centre for Reproductive Medicine at Universitair Ziekenhuis Brussel (UZ Brussel), Brussels, Belgium

Veerle Vloeberghs

Resident gynecologist at the Center for Reproductive Medicine at Universitair Ziekenhuis Brussel (UZ Brussel), Brussels, Belgium

A. Yazdani

Queensland Fertility Group Research Foundation and University of Queensland, Queensland, Australia

Preface

As the range of indications for assisted conception expands and the number and complexity of treatment options available rise, busy clinicians require ready access to information which can guide the management of their patients. Case histories rarely appear now in international journals, but they can serve a very valuable role to illustrate key concepts and options for managing difficult clinical situations in practice.

For this book, four internationally recognized experts in Reproductive Endocrinology and Infertility Medicine have gathered a series of case histories which represent a comprehensive view of the clinical challenges faced in contemporary practice. Written by experienced practicing clinicians, each case describes common and less common presentations, their investigation and management, and also provides the authors' personal reflection on the case and suggested references for further reading.

We thank all the contributors to this book and we hope that our colleagues will find it to be a useful resource.

Abbreviations

ACE	angiotensin-converting enzyme
ACTH	adrenocorticotropic hormone
AFP	alpha-fetoprotein
AI	artificial insemination
AITD	autoimmune thyroid disease
ALT	alanine aminotransferase
AMH	antimüllerian hormone
ANA	antinuclear antibody
APTT	activated partial thromboplastin time
ARDS	acute respiratory distress syndrome
ART	assisted reproductive technology/technologies; assisted reproduction treatment
ASFC	antral follicle count
ASRM	American Society for Reproductive Medicine
AST	aspartate aminotransferase (SGOT)
BEP regimen	bleomycin, etoposide(VP-16), and cisplatin
BHCG	beta-hCG
BMI	body mass index
BP	blood pressure
CBC	complete blood count
CEA	carcinoembryonic antigen
CGH	comparative genomic hybridization
CHB	congenital heart block
CHIPS	the Control of Hypertension in Pregnancy Study
CI	confidence interval
CIN	cervical intraepithelial neoplasia
CKD	chronic kidney disease
CMP	complete metabolic panel
CMV	cytomegalovirus
COC	cumulus–oocyte complex
COH	controlled ovarian hyperstimulation
COS	controlled ovarian stimulation
CRH	corticotropin-releasing hormone
CT	computed tomography
D&C	dilatation and curettage
DHEAS	dehydroepiandrosterone sulfate
DIE	deep infiltrating endometriosis
DVT	deep vein thrombosis
E2	estradiol

ECG	electorcardiography/electorcardiogram
(e)GFR	(estimated) glomerular filtration rate
ENA	extractable nuclear antigen
ER	estrogen receptor
ESHRE	European Society of Human Reproduction and Embryology
FAI	Free Androgen Index
FEC-D	5-fluorouracil–epirubicin–cyclophosphamide followed by docetaxel
FET	frozen embryo transfer cycles
FFP	fresh frozen plasma
FIGO	International Federation of Gynecology and Obstetrics
FSH	follicle-stimulating hormone
FT4	free thyroxine
FXI	factor XI
G-CSF	granulocyte colony-stimulating factor
GCT	glucose challenge test
GDM	gestational diabetes mellitus
GIFT	gamete intrafallopian (tube) transfer
GnRH (GnRHa)	gonadotropin-releasing hormone (agonist)
GV	germinal vesicle
HA	hyaluronic acid
hCG	human chorionic gonadotropin
HCV	hepatitis C virus
HGH	human growth hormone
HIV	human immunodeficiency virus
hMG/HMG	human menopausal gonadotropin
HOS	hypo-osmotic swelling
HP-HMG	highly purified human menopausal gonadotrophin
HP-hMG	high-purity human menopausal gonadotropin
HRT	hormone replacement therapy
HSG	hysterosalpingogram/hysterosalpingography
HTLV	human T-lymphotropic virus
Hycosy	hysterosalpingo-contrast sonography
ICSI	intracytoplasmic sperm injection
IGF1	insulin-like growth factor 1
IM	intramuscular(ly)
IMSI	intracytoplasmic morphologically selected sperm injection
INR	international normalized ratio
ITP	immune thrombocytopenia
IUI	intrauterine insemination
IVF	in vitro fertilization
IVIG	intravenous immunoglobulin
IVM	in vitro maturation
LDH	lactate dehydrogenase
LDR	long down-regulation (protocol)

LH	luteinizing hormone
LLETZ	large loop excisions of transformation zone
LMP	low malignant potential
LMWH	low-molecular-weight heparin
MFM	maternal fetal medicine
MPA	medroxyprogesterone acetate
MRI	magnetic resonance imaging
MTHFR	methylene-tetrahydrofolate reductase
NNT	number needed to treat
NSAID	nonsteroidal anti-inflammatory drug
OCP	oral contraceptive pill
OHSS	ovarian hyperstimulation syndrome
OPU	ovum pick-up
OR	odds ratio
PCO	polycystic ovary
PCOS	polycystic ovary syndrome
PCR	protein/creatinine ratio
PGD	preimplantation genetic diagnosis
PGS	preimplantation genetic screening
PI	pulsatility index
PO	by mouth; orally
POI	premature ovarian insufficiency
PPROM	preterm premature rupture of membranes
PR	progesterone receptor
PRL	prolactin
PT	prothrombin time
PTT	partial thromboplastin time
RCT	randomized controlled trial
rFSH, rec-FSH, rh-FSH	recombinant (human) follicle-stimulating hormone
RI	resistance index
RR	relative risk
SC	subcutaneous(ly)
SCD	sperm chromatin dispersion (test)
SCSA	sperm chromatin structure assay
SGM	surrogate gestational mother
SHBG	sex hormone-binding globulin
SHG	sonohysterogram
SLE	systemic lupus erythematosus
SSRI	selective serotonin reuptake inhibitor
STD	sexually transmitted disease
T2DM	type 2 diabetes mellitus
TG	thyroglobulin
TPO	thyroid peroxidase
TSH	thyroid-stimulating hormone
TVS	transvaginal sonography

USS	ultrasound scan
VDRL	Venereal Disease Research Laboratory (test for syphilis)
VEGF	vascular endothelial growth factor
VTE	venous thromboembolism (VTE)
WBC	white blood cell (count)

Chapter 1

Type 2 diabetes mellitus

Catherine Henry and William M. Hague

Clinical history

Mrs. N. was a 35-year-old process worker who was diagnosed with type 2 diabetes mellitus 2 years previously (random serum glucose 11.4 mmol/L). Both her parents were diabetic. She had two children by a previous partner: the younger was 4 years old, and during that pregnancy the patient experienced gestational diabetes (GDM), which was managed with insulin. Her husband had oligospermia and IVF/ICSI was required. Mrs. N. was maintained on metformin 500 mg tds and daily gliclazide 30 mg: HbA1$_c$ was 8.6%. Her body mass index (BMI) was 31 kg/m^2 and her blood pressure was 130/85 mmHg. She had background minor retinopathy. Urine dipstick analysis showed 1+ protein and serum creatinine 85 μmol/L (upper limit of normal). The couple presented for preconception counseling.

Introduction

Type 2 diabetes mellitus (T2DM) is a common condition that is increasingly diagnosed in younger patients [1, 2]. Its occurrence in women of reproductive age is as much as 20% in some populations [3]. These observations are linked with the rising obesity epidemic in developed countries, associated with more sedentary lifestyles and increased intake of energy-dense food [1, 2].

T2DM is characterized by hyperglycemia secondary to impaired pancreatic beta-cell function and peripheral insulin resistance [1]. End-organ effects, particularly micro- and macrovascular complications during pregnancy may impact both mother and fetus directly and in the longer term [4]. T2DM is associated with increased perinatal mortality, congenital malformations, preeclampsia, birth trauma, and operative delivery [5]. Additionally, the hormonal milieu of pregnancy worsens maternal glycemic control and may accelerate preexisting complications. Although traditionally considered a "less serious" form of diabetes in pregnancy, T2DM is associated with equally poor or worse gestational outcomes than T1DM,with a 4-fold increase in perinatal mortality and a 2-fold increase in congenital malformations. It is crucial that women with T2DM receive effective multidisciplinary care preconception and during pregnancy [1, 2, 4].

Preconception management

Preconception counseling and active management of women with T2DM has been reported to reduce significantly the risk of major congenital malformations[3]. Care focuses on optimizing glycemic control, medication review, identification and treatment of complications, counseling, and reduction of associated risk factors [4, 5]. Effective contraception is advised during the pregnancy-planning period [4]. See Figure 1.1.

History/screening examination

Review of Mrs. N.'s diabetic, obstetric, and personal history was undertaken to identify issues that required correction. Diabetic history must focus on timing of diagnosis, previous and current management, glycemic control, and any active complications [3]. Obstetric history should elucidate previous preeclampsia, intrauterine growth restriction/macrosomia, birth trauma (shoulder dystocia/genital tract injury), and neonatal complications related to diabetes [3]. Modifiable factors include physical inactivity, a high BMI, and poor diet. Nonmodifiable risk factors include ethnicity and a strong family history [5]. GDM carries a 50% risk for the development of T2DM over the next 10 years, so previous care should have incorporated counseling to avert its development. Annual screening of blood glucose is recommended following GDM pregnancy to facilitate early recognition and treatment of T2DM.

Counseling and psychological support

Prepregnancy counseling forewarns about the effects of pregnancy on T2DM and vice versa [2]. It empowers women and promotes uptake of effective management strategies. It should incorporate discussion on the risk of deterioration of diabetic complications, and the potential development of preeclampsia, polyhydramnios, infection, and/or dystocia [4, 5]. Pertinent to this case were concerns regarding deterioration of her sight and renal function, as well as her obesity. Potential fetal complications include miscarriage, stillbirth, and neonatal death [3]. The risk of congenital malformations, including cardiac anomalies, is increased: this is closely related to glycemic control [3, 5]. Strict diabetic control is vital for the long-term health of offspring, as intrauterine programming from exposure to maternal hyperglycemia is associated with higher rates of obesity, metabolic syndrome, and T2DM in later life [1, 5]. Although not all malformations are preventable, careful planning can lessen the potential for many conditions.

T2DM in pregnancy will require heightened monitoring and multidisciplinary involvement [4]. The possibility of preterm or operative delivery (e.g., cesarean section for macrosomia, shoulder dystocia, or previous perineal trauma) should be raised [4]. Discussion should cover increased neonatal risks of hypoglycemia, jaundice, polycythemia, respiratory distress syndrome, hypocalcemia, and the potential for admission to the special care nursery/neonatal intensive care unit [4].

Despite the hazards, it is important to stress that a woman with T2DM can improve the outcome through preventative activities, such as effective blood glucose control and building in gentle exercise.

Medication review

Patients planning pregnancy should undergo medication review to identify potential teratogens [4]. Those pertaining to T2DM include antihyperglycemic, antihypertensive, and lipid-lowering agents [3].

There is long experience with insulin in pregnancy. Its short- and long-term effects (including adverse impacts) have been established over many years [3]. A small number of trials of insulin analog support their safe use in pregnancy [3]. These include insulin lispro and aspart (short-acting analogues) and insulin detemir (long-acting) [3, 5]. Although concerns have been raised that insulin glargine, which has avidity for the insulin-like growth factor receptor-1 and which might cause fetal macrosomia, this has not been confirmed [5].

A basal-bolus regimen, adjusted to fasting and 2-hour postprandial maternal blood glucose, is typically prescribed [4]. Although Mrs. N. might require insulin therapy during pregnancy, given that she had been so treated during her previous pregnancy, her current oral hypoglycemic regimen (metformin and gliclazide) needed to be reviewed prior to conception.

The use of metformin in pregnancy has been assessed in several trials, mainly in patients with polycystic ovary syndrome and in GDM. Though metformin does cross the placenta, there is no increase in congenital abnormalities with its use. Unlike insulin, metformin curtails weight gain and does not carry a significant risk of hypoglycemia. Moreover, by reducing peripheral insulin resistance, its use may allow smaller insulin doses to achieve optimal glycemic control [2]. Limited data suggest no longer-term ill effects on offspring health, cognition, and metabolism [2, 3].

Sulfonylureas are usually avoided in pregnancy due to perceived risks of causing neonatal hypoglycemia, but second-generation agents (e.g., glibenclamide) have been found to be effective and without major adverse events in small trials and cohort studies in the pregnant diabetic population. Although gliclazide may perhaps cross the placenta more easily than glibenclamide, there does not appear to be any significant risk of teratogenesis with these drugs [2].

Angiotensin-converting enzyme (ACE) inhibitors and angiotensin II receptor blockers should generally be ceased during pregnancy: their prolonged use in pregnancy has been associated with abnormalities associated with fetal renal shutdown and anuria, but recent data suggest they are not teratogenic [see Chapter 2 on hypertension]. They may be substituted with methyldopa, labetalol, oxprenolol, nifedipine, clonidine, or prazosin [5]. Atenolol should be ceased in the first trimester due to concerns regarding fetal growth restriction. Diuretics should be avoided unless there is evidence of left ventricular failure. Statins are contraindicated [5].

Glycemic control

Glycemia has a major impact on pregnancy outcomes [3]. It should be stabilized/established prior to conception, as the harmful effects of hyperglycemia during embryogenesis may be more detrimental than the unknown effects of some antihyperglycemic medications [4]. Mrs. N.'s management would optimally include a combination of dietary and lifestyle modifications, insulin, and possibly metformin.

Glycemic control is assessed through patient-monitored fasting and postprandial blood glucose values, together with laboratory measurement of $HbA1_c$ [4]. Mrs. N.'s $HbA1_c$ indicated poor control. Ideally, $HbA1_c$ should be <7% preconception, and preferably within normal limits (<6.1%) [2, 5]. A 1% reduction in $HbA1_c$ correlates with a 40–60% relative risk reduction for congenital malformations [2]. $HbA1_c$ should be monitored each trimester, as a reflection of control over the preceding 8–10 weeks. In pregnancy, $HbA1_c$ normally declines, due to accelerated erythrocyte turnover, particularly in the last two trimesters [5].

During pregnancy, current recommended glucose targets are fasting 4.0–5.5 mmol/L, <8.0 mmol/L at 1 hour postprandial, and <7.0 mmol/L at 2 hours postprandial [5]: it has been suggested that these values are too lax, but there are no randomized trials of treatment to establish either targets in pregnancy or timing of monitoring. Regular blood glucose monitoring is necessary to assist with titration of medication doses. The recommended control of diabetes prepregnancy may take months to achieve, and culturally appropriate education is essential.

Diabetic complications

Patients with diabetes should be screened for complications [5]. Microvascular disease manifests as retinopathy, nephropathy, and neuropathy. These conditions should receive appropriate specialist attention/referral [3].

Diabetic retinopathy (proliferative and nonproliferative) contributes to visual impairment. Pregnancy is a risk factor for acceleration of this condition [3]. Affected women should be reviewed by an ophthalmologist within 12 months before conception [2]. Evidence of proliferative retinopathy warrants treatment (e.g., laser photocoagulation) prior to or during pregnancy [5]. Given Mrs. N.'s mild retinopathy, counseling was considered appropriate regarding the potential for sight deterioration if pregnancy was pursued.

Diabetic nephropathy may also be exacerbated by pregnancy. An assessment for proteinuria and serum creatinine is necessary [2]. Microalbuminuria implies an increased risk for preeclampsia (32–65%), premature delivery (57–91%), and intrauterine growth restriction (12–45%) [3]. Mrs. N.'s proteinuria put her in a higher risk pregnancy category relative to T2DM without proteinuria [5]. Although her serum creatinine was in the upper range of normal, serum creatinine remains within normal limits until substantial deterioration of renal function occurs. A steadily rising creatinine indicates significant renal disease. Nephrology review is recommended for patients whose serum creatinine is >120 mmol/L or whose protein excretion is >2 g/24 hours. Control of glycemia and blood pressure slows disease progression [3].

Neuropathy (autonomic or peripheral) may manifest with orthostatic hypotension, hypoglycemic unawareness, and sensory neuropathy [5]. Pregnant women with these conditions should be advised to be careful when moving from a supine to an erect posture so as to minimize syncope. The risk of hypoglycemic unawareness rises in pregnancy, and these events may be more frequent, particularly in women receiving insulin [4]. Sensory neuropathy is a risk factor for neuropathic ulcers. Weight increase alters the load on the feet. Women should be advised to seek early care if they suspect skin breakdown. Podiatric input may be required.

Macrovascular complications require attention [5]. Some diabetic women will develop cardiovascular disease (e.g., acute coronary syndrome) when cardiology referral is required [2]. A screening ECG is necessary, as well as blood pressure management (particularly in the presence of microalbuminuria and renal impairment) [4]. The target blood pressure is <125/80 mmHg. Mrs. N.'s blood pressure was above that recommended, so it was possible that antihypertensive therapy would be required.

Weight management

Mrs. N. met the BMI criteria for obesity (≥ 30 kg/m^2). Obesity is associated with adverse pregnancy outcomes, additive to those of T2DM [2, 5]. Mrs. N. needed to attempt weight reduction (through exercise and dietary changes), and this would have additional benefit for her diabetes [4]. Any weight loss would be beneficial [2, 3]. Pregnancy weight gain in obese patients is controversial. Some experts recommend restricting weight gain in such women [2, 3].

General advice

T2DM women contemplating pregnancy should be advised to reduce or cease consumption of recreational substances (e.g., alcohol and smoking) and to engage with a management

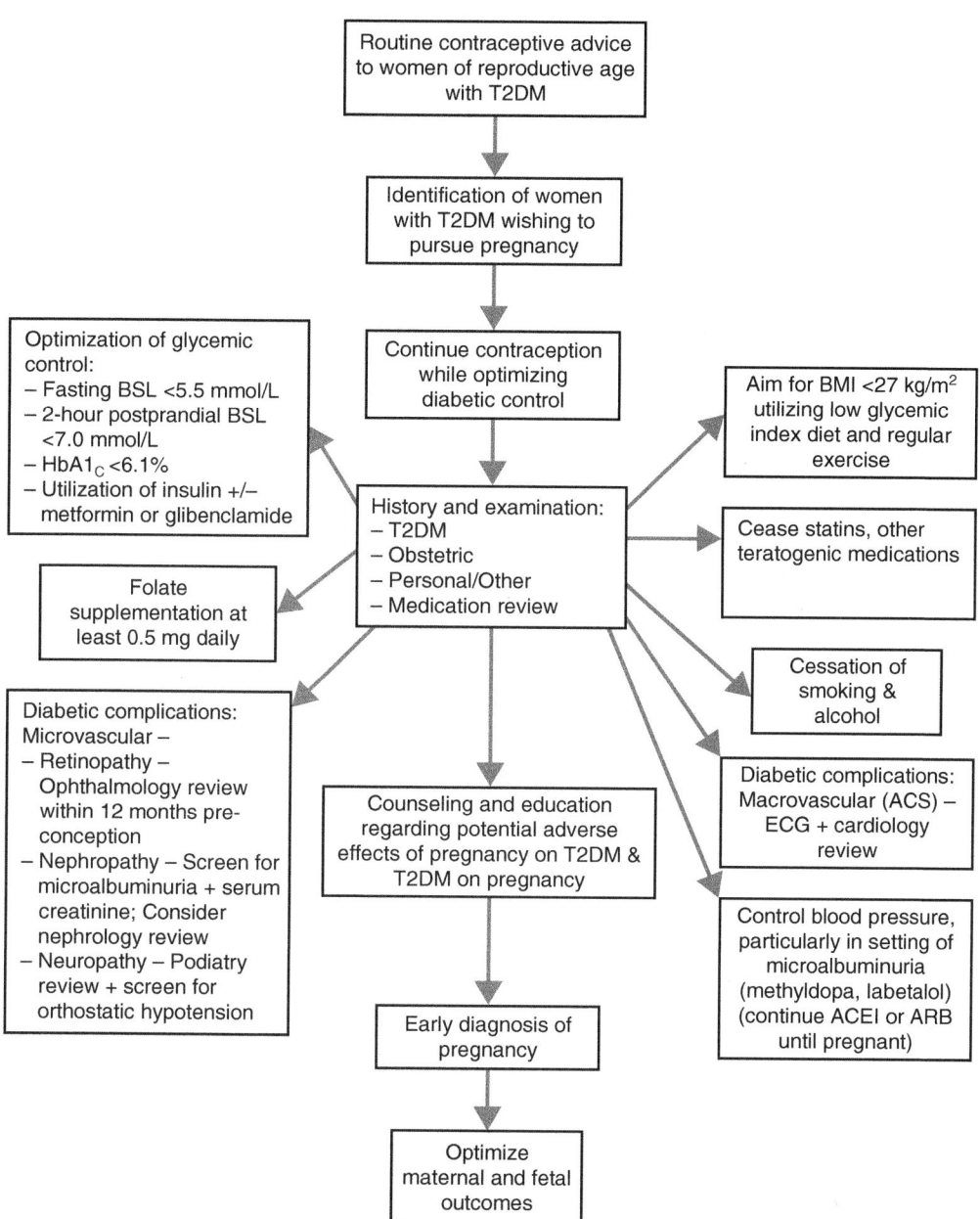

Figure 1.1 A road map for preconception care.

plan to work toward a successful outcome [3]. Preconception folate supplementation until 12 weeks gestation is recommended to prevent neural tube defects [2]. The patient's rubella status should be known and vaccination updated as necessary. Accurate dating of a pregnancy with a late first-trimester ultrasound will guide management throughout the pregnancy, and serum screening should be offered [5]. Pregnant T2DM patients should be encouraged to watch their diet and exercise [2]. A diabetic educator/dietician can advise about the need for low glycemic index foods to stabilize diabetes in a state of flux (i.e., pregnancy) [3]. Dietary habits may be common to the members of the same household. The oligospermia in Mrs. N.'s husband might have been indicative of his personal health issues (e.g., T2DM). Lifestyle changes may well benefit the entire family and improve the fertility of the couple.

Antenatal, intrapartum, and postnatal care

The antenatal, intrapartum, and postnatal care of Mrs. N. will affirm the high-risk nature of any such pregnancy. Close monitoring and tight glycemic control should be continued during and after pregnancy [4]. Assessment for congenital abnormalities and monitoring of fetal growth should be undertaken, with collaboration between obstetricians, obstetric physicians, midwives, endocrinologists, and allied health personnel [5].

Conclusion

T2DM is a major health issue affecting increasing numbers of women of reproductive age. Optimizing glycemic control preconception improves maternal and fetal outcomes with life-long benefits for offspring. Multidisciplinary care is required to attain positive outcomes. This should commence preconception, and continue until the puerperium. Despite Mrs. N.'s suboptimal diabetic management, alterations to therapy can improve significantly both her health and that of any offspring. Lifestyle modifications may also have benefits for the family.

References

1. Nolan CJ, Damm P, Prentki M. Type 2 diabetes across generations: from pathophysiology to prevention and management. *Lancet* 2011; **378**: 169–81.

2. Temple R, Murphy H. Type 2 diabetes in pregnancy – An increasing problem. *Best Practice & Research Clinical Endocrinology & Metabolism* 2010; **24**: 591–603.

3. McCance DR. Pregnancy and diabetes. *Best Practice & Research Clinical Endocrinology & Metabolism* 2011; **25**: 945–58.

4. Mahmud M, Mazza D. Preconception care of women with diabetes: a review of current guideline recommendations. *BMC Women's Health* 2010; **10**: 5 Available from: http://www.biomedcentral.com/1472-6874/10/5.

5. McElduff A, Cheung NW, McIntyre HD, Lagstrom JA, Oats JJN, Ross GP, Simmons D, Walters BNJ, Wein P. The Australasian Diabetes in Pregnancy Society consensus guidelines for the management of type 1 and type 2 diabetes in relation to pregnancy. *Medical Journal of Australia* 2005; **183**: 373–7.

Chapter

2

A woman with hypertension

Mark R. Morton and William M. Hague

Clinical history

Ms. B. was a 28-year-old teacher from the northern suburbs of the metropolis, who had never been pregnant, despite 2 years of unprotected intercourse, regular ovulatory menses, and a 38-year-old partner with three previous paternities. She was diagnosed with hypertension while taking the combined oral contraceptive pill and remained hypertensive despite coming off the pill. Her father was hypertensive and had a stroke in his sixties. Her current treatment included irbesartan 150 mg daily. On examination, she was anxious. Blood pressure was 150/90 mmHg. Eyes were normal. Urine dipstick showed a trace of protein. Electrolytes, blood glucose, and renal function were normal.

What further investigations should be considered?

The family history of hypertension and cerebrovascular disease suggests a diagnosis of essential hypertension. However, secondary causes of hypertension should also be considered, particularly renal disease, which can also be familial. The urine dipstick result is probably not significant, but it would be worth quantifying any proteinuria with a urinary microalbumin test, which can be measured on a spot urine. The presence of significant urinary albumin would support a diagnosis of underlying renal disease or renal damage from long-standing hypertension. A renal ultrasound should be performed to assess renal size and to look for any renal scarring. Renal artery stenosis due to fibromuscular dysplasia is a rare secondary cause of renovascular hypertension, but can occur in young women. This can sometimes be diagnosed on renal artery Doppler studies, but computed tomography (CT) or magnetic resonance (MR) angiography are more sensitive investigations for renal artery stenosis.

Hypertension in a young person, especially if severe, can be due to a coarctation of the aorta, so the femoral pulses should be checked and compared to the radial pulses to see whether there is any radio-femoral delay.

Hypertension with symptoms, such as abdominal pain, palpitations, sweating, and anxiety, could indicate a pheochromocytoma. This is an epinephrine (adrenaline)- and/or norepinephrine (noradrenaline)-secreting tumor, usually of the adrenal gland. Ten percent of such tumors can be extra-adrenal and 10% are malignant. Although this is a very rare cause of secondary hypertension, if it is missed in pregnancy the consequences can be catastrophic for both the mother and fetus. A 24-hour urine collection for urinary catecholamines is an appropriate screening test for pheochromocytoma. (It is important to collect the urine into a container with added acid to minimize spontaneous degradation of any catecholamine present.)

Not infrequently, the finding of elevated blood pressure in the clinic may be related to anxiety rather than to true chronic hypertension. Ambulatory 24-hour blood pressure monitoring is increasingly being used to identify patients with "white-coat" hypertension. Women with "white-coat" hypertension do have better outcomes in pregnancy than those with true chronic hypertension, but despite the label they are still at slightly increased risk of developing hypertensive disorders of pregnancy.

Preexisting hypertension for any reason is a risk factor for the subsequent development of preeclampsia. The risk of developing preeclampsia is increased 5-fold in women with prior hypertension. Ms. B. should therefore be counseled regarding the possibility of pre-eclampsia and associated intrauterine growth restriction. These risks are further increased in women undergoing assisted reproduction, particularly if the woman is obese. Multifetal pregnancy also compounds the risk, and every effort should be made to ensure a singleton pregnancy in the hypertensive woman undergoing assisted reproductive technology.

Should she be given agents to prevent preeclampsia?

Many studies have been performed to identify agents that might prevent preeclampsia, particularly in high-risk women. Aspirin, calcium, and antioxidant vitamins have been the most extensively studied.

A Cochrane review found that use of antiplatelet agents, in particular aspirin at a dose of 75–150 mg/day, gives a small but significant reduction (0.83: 95% confidence interval [CI] 0.77 to 0.89) in the relative risk of developing preeclampsia, as well as a reduction in the risk of perinatal mortality (0.86: 95% CI 0.76 to 0.98). In high-risk women, only 19 need to be treated to prevent one case of preeclampsia. There is a halving of the risk when treatment is started before 16 weeks gestation. Meta-analysis of individual patient data from the Cochrane review did not show any difference in risk reduction for the presence of chronic hypertension. Current guidelines recommend that aspirin should be commenced after 12 weeks gestation and before 20 weeks gestation in women with moderate or high risk of developing preeclampsia. Low-dose aspirin is considered safe in pregnancy: it does not increase the rates of antepartum or postpartum hemorrhage or of placental abruption.

Calcium supplementation of at least 1 gram per day during pregnancy can reduce the overall risk of developing preeclampsia (RR 0.65: 95% CI 0.53 to 0.81). This relative risk reduction is greatest in populations with poor dietary calcium intake and is less marked in populations that have adequate dietary calcium. Current guidelines recommend that calcium supplements should be given to women with poor dietary calcium intake and to those at high risk of preeclampsia.

Randomized controlled trials of the antioxidants vitamin C and vitamin E have failed to show any benefit in preventing preeclampsia or improving pregnancy outcomes. Observational data suggest that continuing folic acid supplements beyond the end of the first trimester is associated with a lower risk of preeclampsia: a large international RCT is currently in progress to assess this further.

If she is planning a pregnancy, does her antihypertensive treatment need to be changed?

Use of angiotensin-converting enzyme (ACE) inhibitors in the second and third trimesters of pregnancy is contraindicated because of an increased risk of adverse fetal outcomes.

Exposed fetuses are at increased risk of oligohydramnios, intrauterine growth restriction, hypocalvaria, renal dysplasia, and death. It is thought that a functioning renin–angiotensin system is required for the development of the fetal kidney. Because of a similar mechanism of action, angiotensin II receptor antagonists, such as irbesartan, are also contraindicated in the second and third trimesters.

The use of ACE inhibitors or angiotensin II receptor antagonists in the first trimester was also previously considered to be undesirable. However, recent population-based cohort studies and a meta-analysis have challenged this view.

In 2006, a cohort study of 29 507 births reported an increase in congenital malformations in the 209 infants that had been exposed to ACE inhibitors in the first trimester. Compared with fetuses who had had no exposure to antihypertensive agents in the first trimester, those exposed to ACE inhibitors had a 2.7-fold increase in congenital malformations, mainly of the cardiovascular and central nervous systems [1]. However, a more recent and much larger cohort study of 465 754 mother–infant pairs, in which 400 infants were exposed to ACE inhibitors, found only a nonsignificant 20% increased risk of any congenital malformation [2]. Furthermore, infants exposed to any antihypertensive agent in the first trimester, as well as infants of women who had hypertension but who did not take antihypertensive medication in the first trimester, had similar increased rates of congenital malformations. The apparent increased risk of congenital malformations in women with hypertension seems likely to be associated with the hypertension itself rather than the antihypertensive drugs.

A meta-analysis performed in 2011 of five observational cohort studies of 786 exposed infants and over one million controls concluded that first-trimester exposure to ACE inhibitors and angiotensin II receptor blockers was not associated with an elevated risk of major malformations compared with exposure to other antihypertensive agents [3]. Therefore, if Ms. B. needs antihypertensive treatment, it will be reasonable to continue the angiotensin receptor blocker until a pregnancy is confirmed.

Does she need to continue her antihypertensive agent?

In women with mild hypertension controlled on a single antihypertensive agent, given the natural fall in blood pressure in the first trimester, it is reasonable once a pregnancy is confirmed to cease the antihypertensive agent and to monitor the blood pressure. The levels of blood pressure at which hypertension in pregnancy should be treated are controversial. A Cochrane review has concluded that it is unclear whether the treatment of mild to moderate hypertension in pregnancy is worthwhile [4]. Hypertension treatment in pregnancy will halve the risk of a woman having one or more episodes of severe hypertension. Between 8 and 13 pregnant women will need to be treated with an antihypertensive drug to prevent one episode of severe hypertension. There are insufficient data to determine whether this provides substantial maternal benefits or improves fetal or neonatal outcomes. Overtreatment of blood pressure in pregnancy may impair utero-placental perfusion, leading to fetal growth restriction and adverse fetal outcomes. More data are needed and it is hoped that the results from the Control of Hypertension in Pregnancy Study (CHIPS), a multicenter randomized controlled trial examining nonsevere nonproteinuric hypertension in pregnancy that has recently completed recruitment, will provide much-needed guidance on appropriate targets for blood pressure control in pregnancy [5]. Until then, the question whether "less tight" control or "tight" control of blood pressure in pregnancy increases or decreases the likelihood of pregnancy loss or high-level neonatal care remains moot.

What antihypertensive agent should be used?

A Cochrane review of antihypertensive treatment in pregnancy failed to find that any particular drug was superior to any other [4]. Consensus guidelines have been published in the United Kingdom, Canada, United States, Australia, and New Zealand. The three most commonly used antihypertensive drugs used in pregnancy are labetalol, methyldopa, and nifedipine.

Labetalol is a competitive α_1- and nonselective β-adrenoreceptor blocker. The combined α- and β-blockade contributes to the blood pressure lowering effect, while the β-blocking properties prevent the reflex tachycardia that can occur with α-blocking agents. Chronic administration results in considerable reduction in blood pressure and peripheral resistance and a less-marked reduction in heart rate and cardiac output. Labetalol is a reasonable choice for treatment of hypertension in each trimester of pregnancy. An intravenous formulation is available for treatment of hypertensive emergencies in pregnancy. Very low amounts of the drug are excreted in breast milk and it is considered safe to use while breast feeding.

Methyldopa was developed in the 1950s to block the action of the enzyme dopa-decarboxylase, thereby preventing the formation of norepinephrine (noradrenaline). However, its active metabolite α-methylnorepinephrine stimulates the central α_2 receptors in the brainstem, resulting in its blood pressure-lowering effect. It is considered safe to use in each trimester of pregnancy. Sedation and tiredness are common side effects which can limit its usefulness, particularly if larger doses are needed to control blood pressure. It is safe to use while breast-feeding but it can exacerbate depression in the postnatal period. It is one of the few drugs that have any long-term outcome data in relation to the offspring exposed during pregnancy. A study published in 1982 looking at 195 children followed up to age 7 years after exposure to methyldopa used for treatment of hypertension in pregnancy did not find any adverse effects.

Nifedipine is a dihydropyridine calcium channel blocker. Calcium channel blockers cause interference with the entry of calcium ions into cells by blocking voltage-gated calcium channels in cardiac and smooth-muscle cells. This results in arterial vasodilatation and direct effects on cardiac conduction and contractility. It is considered safe to use in each trimester of pregnancy. Slow-release formulations can be used for treatment of chronic hypertension in pregnancy, while quick-acting versions are valuable for treatment of hypertensive emergencies. Side effects include headache, flushing, ankle edema, and a reflex tachycardia. Only small amounts of drug are excreted in breast milk and it is considered safe to give to nursing mothers. Nifedipine is also used as a tocolytic agent. Interestingly, there does not appear to be a marked effect on blood pressure when used in the normotensive woman in preterm labor.

Other antihypertensive agents that have been used to manage chronic hypertension in pregnancy include hydralazine, prazosin, and clonidine. Diuretics have been employed as fourth-line agents in difficult chronic hypertension, although there are concerns about potential reductions in circulating plasma volume, which might reduce placental blood flow in preeclampsia, as well as causing hyperuricemia, making assessment of superimposed preeclampsia more difficult [6].

References

1. Cooper WO, Hernandez-Diaz S, Arbogast PG *et al*. Major congenital malformations after first trimester exposure to ACE inhibitors. *N Engl J Med* 2006; **354**: 2443–51.

2. Li DK, Yang C, Andrade S, Tavares V, Ferber JR. Maternal exposure to angiotensin converting enzyme inhibitors in the first trimester and risk of malformations in offspring: a retrospective cohort study. *BMJ* 2011; **343**: d5931.

3. Walfisch A, Al-maawali A, Moretti ME, Nickel C, Koren G. Teratogenicity of angiotensin converting enzyme inhibitors or receptor blockers. *J Obstet Gynecol* 2011; **31**: 465–72.

4. Abalos E, Duley L, Steyn DW, Henderson-Smart DJ. Antihypertensive drug therapy for mild to moderate hypertension during pregnancy. *Cochrane Database Syst Rev* 2007; (1): CD002252. DOI: 10.1002/14651858.CD002252.pub2

5. Magee LA, von Dadelszen P, Chan S *et al*. The Control of Hypertension In Pregnancy Study pilot trial. *BJOGgyneco* 2007; **114**: 770, e13–20.

6. Duley L, Henderson-Smart DJ, Meher S, King JF. Antiplatelet agents for preventing pre-eclampsia and its complications. *Cochrane Database Syst Rev* 2007; (2): CD004659. DOI: 10.1002/14651858.CD004659.pub2

Chapter

3

Increased risk of venous thromboembolism (VTE)

Nick S. Macklon

Clinical fertility history

A 36-year-old nulligravid woman with a 3-year history of primary infertility, previously diagnosed with polycystic ovary syndrome presented for IVF treatment after failure to conceive with ovulation induction.

General medical, family, and social history

The patient had no previous medical history of note, and specifically, no previous history of venous thromboembolism (VTE). She was, however, obese, with a sedentary lifestyle. Previous attempts to lose weight had been only transiently successful. She continued to smoke 10–15 cigarettes a day, as she had for many years.

Examination findings

On examination her BMI was 36, she had mild hirsutism and normal external genitalia. No other abnormalities were evident.

Fertility investigations

Early follicular phase endocrinology was consistent with WHO type 2 anovulation, with an FSH level of 6.7 IU/L, LH of 11 IU/L, and an estradiol of 320 pmol/L. Her antimüllerian hormone (AMH) level was 32 pmol/L. She had both clinical and biochemical evidence of hyperandrogenism. On transvaginal ultrasound, her ovaries were visible and were observed to be polycystic. No other abnormalities of her internal genitalia were detected.

A previous hysterosalpingo-contrast sonography (Hycosy) examination had demonstrated tubal patency. Her partner, who was moderately overweight and a light smoker, was otherwise well, with no past history of note. Semen analysis parameters were within the normal range.

Other clinical investigations

A fasting glucose level was within the normal range. The patient presented with a number of risk factors for developing DVT in association with IVF treatment and pregnancy (Table 3.1), and investigations to exclude a thrombophilia were performed. Tests for the most common acquired thrombophilias: lupus anticoagulant and anticardiolipin were negative, and the patient was found to have no evidence of the congenital thrombophilias associated with deficiency of protein C, protein S, or antithrombin, or genetic mutations in the procoagulant factors prothrombin G20210A or methylene-tetrahydrofolate reductase (MTHFR) genes.

Table 3.1 Risk factors for venous thromboembolism present in the patient

Age >35 years
BMI >30 kg/m²
Heavy smoker
Sedentary lifestyle
Polycystic ovary syndrome (PCOS) and therefore at greater risk of developing ovarian hyperstimulation syndrome (OHSS)

However, the patient was found to be heterozygous for the Factor V Leiden mutation. Her blood count parameters, including platelets, were normal.

Diagnosis

Primary anovulatory infertility resistant to ovulation induction in an obese woman with polycystic ovary syndrome (PCOS), who smoked and was revealed to be heterozygotic for Factor V Leiden mutation.

Action plan

The patient and her partner were successfully advised to give up smoking prior to starting IVF treatment. Given the risk factors present for developing VTE, the following further steps were taken:

1. She was fitted with compression stockings before starting ovarian stimulation.
2. A milder ovarian stimulation regimen was employed, starting with 150 IU rec FSH on cycle day, and co-treatment with a GnRH antagonist from stimulation day 5 to prevent premature luteinization.
3. Twenty-four hours after oocyte pickup, she commenced daily treatment with subcutaneous enoxaparin 40 mg per day, with the aim of continuing this up to 10 weeks gestation if she conceived.
4. She underwent transfer of a single embryo.
5. For luteal phase support she received vaginal micronized progesterone pessaries, 200 mg three times a day, in order to reduce the risk of developing OHSS associated with using hCG for luteal support.

Outcome

The patient conceived a singleton intrauterine pregnancy. During the luteal phase and early pregnancy she was seen regularly to exclude clinical signs of ovarian hyperstimulation syndrome (OHSS). After two weeks on enoxaparin, a platelet count excluded heparin-induced thrombocytopenia.

During her scan at 7 weeks to confirm ongoing pregnancy, she reported left-sided discomfort in the neck. On examination there was no evidence of swelling. However, given the association reported between IVF and the development of upper extremity ultrasound, an ultrasound of the jugular vein was performed. This showed no evidence of VTE. She continued into an otherwise uncomplicated pregnancy, stopping enoxaparin at 10 weeks, and delivered a healthy boy at 38 weeks gestation by cesarean section.

General remarks

VTE is a rare complication of IVF, with a reported incidence of 0.08–0.11% of treatment cycles (Chan and Ginsberg 2006). However, IVF treatment is a known risk factor, since ovarian stimulation, and in particular hCG triggering is known to induce prothrombotic changes in clotting factor profiles. The short- and long-term morbidity of VTE is significant and therefore all patients attending for IVF should undergo a risk assessment for VTE before starting treatment. This patient had no previous history of VTE, but presented with a number of risk factors for developing thrombotic complications from IVF treatment, as shown in Table 3.1. In themselves these can be considered sufficient risk factors to require exclusion of a thrombophilia as part of risk assessment for deep venous thrombosis (Macklon 2014). The presented patient was revealed to be heterozygous for Factor V Leiden mutation, which is the most common thrombophilia, with a prevalence of 2–7% in the European population (Nelson and Greer, 2009). The presence of a heterozygous Factor V Leiden mutation is estimated to increase the risk of VTE in pregnancy by a factor of almost 10, rising to 35 when the patient is homozygous for the mutation (Robertson et al. 2006) The combination of risk factors merited taking the steps described to prevent VTE.

The use of low-dose FSH with GnRH antagonist rather than GnRH agonist co-treatment has been shown to reduce the risk of developing OHSS (Al-Inany et al, 2011), and since this is a major risk factor for VTE, consideration of an appropriate stimulation and luteal support regimen was important.

When VTE occurs in association with IVF it is most commonly some weeks after treatment. Therefore thromboprophylaxis should extend up to 10 weeks gestation.

This should consist of compression stockings and low-molecular-weight heparin. It is usually advised to commence thromboprophylaxis at the start of ovarian stimulation (Nelson and Greer 2009). While bleeding complications associated with oocyte retrieval procedures are rare (Yinon et al. 2006), some advocate withholding heparin for 24 hours on the day of oocyte pickup. The procoagulant effects of ovarian stimulation are far more marked following triggering of final oocyte maturation with hCG (Macklon 2014), and if there is a concern regarding bleeding complications then it is reasonable to delay starting heparin thromboprophylaxis treatment until 24 hours after oocyte pickup.

In the presented case, both the IVF treatment and thromboprophylaxis were successful. However, during a routine ultrasound scan at 7 weeks gestation, the patient described neck symptoms which merited investigation, as a number of cases of late, upper extremity VTE have been reported after IVF, even in women receiving thromboprophylaxis (Chan and Ginsberg 2006). Indeed the relative prevalence of this location for VTE appears to be higher after IVF. The mechanism behind this remains unclear, but it has been proposed that peritoneal fluid high in estradiol concentrations produced by the stimulated ovaries enters the lymph system and is transported via the thoracic and lymphatic ducts to the chest, where it drains into the junction of the subclavian vein and jugular veins, causing local procoagulant conditions (Bauersachs et al. 2007).

In the presented case however, an ultrasound scan of her neck veins excluded a VTE, and her symptoms resolved spontaneously. Thromboprophylaxis was stopped at 10 weeks gestation, and the patient went on to deliver at term by cesarean section, for which she received postpartum thromboprophylaxis.

References

Al-Inany HG, Youssef MA, Aboulghar M, Broekmans F, Sterrenburg M, Smit J, Abou-Setta AM. Gonadotropin-releasing hormone antagonists for assisted reproductive technology. *Cochrane Database Syst Rev* 2011; (**5**): CD001750.

Bauersachs RM, Manolopoulos K, Hoppe I, Arin MJ, Schleussner E. More on: the 'ART' behind the clot: solving the mystery. *J Thromb Haemost* 2007; **5**: 438–9.

Chan WS, Ginsberg JS. A review of upper extremity deep vein thrombosis in pregnancy: unmasking the 'ART' behind the clot. *J Thromb Haemost* 2006; **4**:1673–7.

Macklon NS; The patient at risk of thromboembolic disease. In: Macklon NS (Ed.) *IVF in the Medically Complicated Patient.* 2nd edition. London: Taylor and Francis; 2014.

Nelson S, Greer IA. The patient at risk from thrombosis and bleeding disorders. In: Macklon NS, Greer AI, Steegers EAP (Eds.). *Textbook of Periconceptional Medicine.* London: Informa; 2009:121–36.

Robertson L, Wu O, Langthorne P, Twaddle S, Clark P, Lowe GD, Greaves M, Brenkel I, Regan L, Greer IA. Thrombophilia in pregnancy: a systematic review. *Br J Haematol* 2006;**132**:171–96.

Yinon Y, Pauzner R, Dulitsky M, Elizur SE, Dor J, Shulman A. Safety of IVF under anticoagulant therapy in patients at risk of thrombo-embolic events. *Reprod Biomed Online* 2006;**12**:354–8.

Chapter 4

Assisted reproduction in a subfertile couple with serodiscordant HIV infection

S. McDowell, B. Kroon, and A. Yazdani

Clinical fertility history

Mrs. S. (31 years old) and Mr. S. (34 years old) were a Cambodian couple who presented with infertility after a 2-year history of intermittent unprotected intercourse. Mr. S. had been diagnosed with human immunodeficiency virus type 1 infection (HIV) 8 years earlier. Aware of the risks of HIV transmission the couple had elected to time unprotected intercourse to the days around supposed ovulation, while at other times in the cycle they used condoms. He was on antiviral medication. Mrs. S. had regular HIV serology performed, which was consistently negative.

General medical, family, and social history:

Mrs. S. was fit and well, a nonsmoker, and with no medical or surgical history of note. Menstrual cycles were regular every 28 days, with moderate dysmenorrhea on days 1–3 of the cycle. Menstrual flow was normal. She had no history of sexually transmitted infections and had ceased the combined oral contraceptive pill 2 years previously to use condoms most of the month.

Mr. S. was diagnosed with HIV and pulmonary tuberculosis following emigration 9 years earlier. The tuberculosis was treated effectively and he was asymptomatic of HIV infection at the time of presentation. He was taking highly active antiretroviral treatment (efavirenz, emtricitabine, tenofovir) under the care of the local public hospital infectious disease unit. Most recent bloods showed normal CD4 count (460 cells/mm^3) and undetectable serum HIV viral load on polymerase chain reaction.

Examination findings

Mrs. S. weighed 63 kg with a body mass index of 23.0 kg/m^2. Mr. S. weighed 70 kg with a body mass index of 21.0 kg/m^2. Examination was normal for both. Female pelvic examination was unremarkable, and male genital examination revealed a normal phallus and normal testicular volumes.

Fertility investigations

Mrs. S. had a mid-luteal progesterone consistent with previous ovulation and an antimüllerian hormone (AMH) of 14.5 pmol/L (normal for her age). HIV enzyme immunoassay and serological tests for hepatitis B and hepatitis C were negative. She was rubella and varicella immune and had a normal TSH and vitamin D. Ultrasound scan showed a normal anteverted uterus, normal ovaries, and a combined antral follicle count of 11.

Mr. S.'s semen analysis showed concentration of 45 million/mL, total sperm motility 60%, and sperm morphology 2%. Repeat semen analysis was unchanged. Hepatitis B and hepatitis C serology were negative.

Other clinical investigations

Given the history of dysmenorrhea in the presence of subfertility, Mrs. S. was offered a laparoscopy, hysteroscopy, and tubal dye studies. Laparoscopy revealed stage 1 endometriosis (American Society of Reproductive Medicine revised classification), which was excised. Hysteroscopy was unremarkable and fallopian tubes were patent.

Diagnosis

Two years of primary infertility likely related to teratozoospermia and mild endometriosis, in the presence of serodiscordant HIV infection (male partner HIV positive).

Action plan

Reproductive options and associated risks were outlined and in view of serodiscordant HIV and teratozoospermia, in vitro fertilization (IVF) with intracytoplasmic sperm injection (ICSI) was recommended. Prior to IVF, an aliquot of semen underwent testing for HIV RNA (viral load) and when it was found to be negative the remainder of the semen was washed and cryopreserved. A GnRH antagonist stimulation protocol was selected with a recombinant follicle-stimulating hormone (FSH) dose of 150 IU daily.

Outcome

HIV viral load was undetectable in the semen and four ampoules were cryopreserved. Seven oocytes were retrieved and six were fertilized following ICSI. A single blastocyst transfer was performed and two blastocysts were cryopreserved in a designated tank. Serum BhCG was positive 12 days post oocyte retrieval and subsequent transvaginal ultrasound scan at 7 weeks gestational age showed a single viable intrauterine pregnancy. HIV serology remained negative throughout pregnancy, during which condom use was maintained.

General remarks

Managed with long-term suppressive therapy, HIV infection can now be considered a chronic controllable disease. An increasing number of HIV-infected couples will present for infertility investigation and management. In couples with serodiscordant HIV infection, management is focused on risk minimization.

In serodiscordant couples where the woman is HIV positive, artificial insemination (AI) and IVF greatly minimize the risk of HIV transmission. A single act of unprotected vaginal intercourse carries of 0.05% risk of HIV transmission to the man [1].

In HIV-positive men, mature spermatozoa do not express CD4 receptors or co-receptors that are needed for HIV binding. As such, the HIV virus is present in seminal secretions but not in spermatozoa themselves. In couples where the man is HIV positive a single act of unprotected intercourse carries a 0.1% risk of disease transmission to the woman [1]. The risk of HIV transmission to the female partner is considered slight if the man is compliant with treatment, has no other infections, has a plasma viral load of less than 50 copies/mL, and unprotected vaginal intercourse is limited to the time of ovulation. If serum viral load is greater than 50 copies/mL but seminal viral load is undetectable, timed unprotected intercourse can still be considered.

Many couples and practitioners will consider this risk unacceptable and utilize sperm washing [2]. Spermatozoa are separated from seminal fluid and analyzed for viral load. Samples negative for HIV RNA can be used for AI or IVF. To date, there are no reported cases of female infection following sperm washing. IVF and ICSI should be reserved for standard clinical indications. ICSI has not been shown to reduce risks of HIV transmission [3].

The majority of HIV-positive men have semen parameters within the normal range. There is, however, a significant negative correlation with all semen parameters as general health and CD4 count deteriorate.

Other options for serodiscordant HIV couples include the use of donor sperm and adoption. Pre- and postexposure prophylactic antiretroviral therapy has been postulated as a means to reduce HIV transmission [4,5]. The risk appears to be reduced but not eliminated and this method is not currently recommended until further evidence is available.

Pregnancy does not appear to increase the risk of progression of disease in asymptomatic HIV-positive women. The risk of miscarriage, preterm delivery, and fetal growth restriction may be increased; however, this is likely related to maternal disease rather than HIV infection. To reduce the risk of vertical transmission, antiretroviral treatment is commonly administered. Planned vaginal delivery is not recommended in women with a positive HIV viral load.

References

1. Powers K, Poole C, Pettifor A, Cohen M. Rethinking the heterosexual infectivity of HIV-1: a systematic review and meta-analysis. *Lancet Infect Dis* 2008; **8**(9): 553.

2. Sauer M. Sperm washing techniques address the fertility needs of HIV-seropositive men: a clinical review. *Reprod BioMedicine Online* 2005; **10**(1): 135–40.

3. Garrido N, Meseguer M, Bellver J *et al.* Report of the results of a 2 year programme of sperm wash and ICSI treatment for human immunodeficiency virus and hepatitis C virus serodiscordant couples. *Hum Reprod* 2004; **19**: 2581.

4. Cohen M *et al.* Prevention of HIV-1 infection with early antiretroviral therapy. *N Engl J Med* 2011; **365**(6): 493.

5. Katz M, Gerberding J. The care of persons with recent sexual exposure to HIV. *Ann Intern Med* 1998; **128**(4): 306.

Chapter 5

A woman with renal impairment

Shilpa Jesudason and William M. Hague

Clinical history

Ms. M. was a 25-year-old Filipino migrant, who had been trying to conceive for a year to an older Australian partner, who had 2 previous children. She reported regular menses. Her mother had some kind of kidney problem. Her blood pressure was normal. Urine dipstick showed 3+ protein. Routine investigations showed increased serum creatinine (150 μmol/L) and a normal blood picture. Urine microscopy demonstrated no casts or cells, and culture showed no growth.

Case discussion

Ms. M. was likely to have chronic kidney disease (CKD), which might affect her fertility and future health, and which would increase her risk of adverse pregnancy outcomes. She therefore required further workup and counseling before conception or assisted reproduction.

The features of CKD in this patient included:

1. Reduced renal function, as assessed by creatinine and estimated glomerular filtration rate (eGFR). Using the CKD-EPI formula, Ms. M.'s eGFR was 41 mL/min/1.73 m², indicating stage 3 CKD.
2. Overt (dipstick positive) proteinuria of +3 severity.
3. The duration of these abnormalities is important, to differentiate an acute renal problem from chronic kidney disease, where the duration is usually >3 months.
4. The absence of hypertension was reassuring. Hypertension is common in CKD due to disturbed renal regulation of blood pressure.
5. The absence of urinary cells, particularly dysmorphic red blood cells (indicating glomerular hematuria), and absence of tubular casts (tubular-shaped structures consisting of cells or proteins from glomerular damage or inflammation) made glomerulonephritis less likely, though not excluded.
6. Heavy proteinuria indicates significant kidney damage and is a feature of many renal diseases.
7. The urine culture did not show current infection. The presence of recurrent urinary tract infection (particularly in childhood) may suggest reflux nephropathy. Reflux nephropathy may present with a family history of renal problems in first-degree female relatives, CKD, proteinuria, and commonly hypertension.
8. The differential diagnosis was quite wide and further investigations are necessary to establish the cause of the renal abnormalities. Basic investigations should include quantification of proteinuria, assessment of urine sediment and microscopy, blood biochemistry, and renal imaging with ultrasound.

9. Referral to a nephrologist for further investigation including possible renal biopsy would be warranted in a young woman with significant proteinuria and abnormal renal function.

Background

The physiological changes of pregnancy place the kidneys under considerable stress. Renal perfusion and GFR increase early in the first trimester by 50–60%, leading to a rise in creatinine clearance, hyperfiltration, and increased protein excretion. There are altered hemodynamics, with salt and water retention, and renin–angiotensin system activation. Total renal volume increases and urinary tract dilatation occurs, due to the effects of progesterone and mechanical compression.

Consequently, silent CKD may be unmasked in pregnancy, or existing CKD may worsen. Women with CKD require counseling before pregnancy and may require specialized management during pregnancy. It is important to identify women with CKD as early as possible, ideally before conception, to allow one to provide prepregnancy counseling, perform appropriate investigations, optimize medical management, and decide on the appropriate timing of conception for the best maternal and fetal outcomes.

CKD affects 3–5% of women of child-bearing age. However, severe CKD (stage 4–5) in pregnancy is very uncommon, due to the markedly reduced fertility in this population. The causes of CKD in this age group are most commonly glomerulonephritis (including IgA nephropathy, lupus nephritis, hereditary disorders, and other rarer conditions), polycystic kidney disease, and reflux nephropathy. Diabetic and ischemic nephropathy are leading causes of CKD overall but are less common in this age group.

Women with CKD identified prepregnancy or in pregnancy should be further evaluated for the degree of CKD and underlying cause of CKD, as this will have an impact on the outcome of pregnancy.

Diagnosis of chronic kidney disease

CKD is divided into five stages according to eGFR and urine/structural abnormalities (Table 5.1). CKD occurs when eGFR is <60 mL/min/1.73 m², or if there is other evidence of renal disease, such as pathological or structural damage, micro- or macro-albuminuria, or glomerular hematuria. Estimated GFR and urine assessment for albuminuria/proteinuria in combination are the key tests for the detection of CKD.

Glomerular filtration rate

Glomerular filtration rate (GFR) may be estimated by a number of equations – in Australia, laboratories routinely report eGFR based on the MDRD formula or more recently the CKD-EPI formula. These formulae provide a valid estimate of GFR in prepregnancy women, and correlate well with measured GFR, particularly when GFR is <60 mL/min. However, once pregnancy is established, estimated GFR calculations are less reliable, and have not been validated in the pregnant population. Hyperfiltration and hemodilution due to the physiological changes of pregnancy will both affect serum creatinine, which is the main parameter in all eGFR equations.

Proteinuria

Early morning urine albumin/creatinine ratio is recommended to screen for albuminuria associated with CKD [1], and it may be elevated even if urine dipstick is negative. Random

Table 5.1 Stages of CKD [2]

CKD stage	GFR (mL/min/1.73 m² BSAª)	
Stage 1	>90	Only considered to be CKD if other abnormalities are also present
Stage 2	60–89	
Stage 3a	45–59	
Stage 3b	30–44	
Stage 4	15–29	
Stage 5	<15	

ª Body surface area.

urine protein/creatinine ratio (PCR) is the next step in assessing the degree of proteinuria in women with overt proteinuria (positive dipstick readings). If significant proteinuria is evident on urine PCR, further quantification with a timed urine collection is useful, to establish whether there is subnephrotic range (<3 g/day protein excretion) or nephrotic range (>3 g/day protein excretion). In pregnancy, urine dipstick for protein can assist in excluding women without significant proteinuria. In those with positive urine dipstick, urine PCR should be performed. The urine PCR has been well validated in pregnancy as a surrogate for formal 24-hour urine collections, which are inconvenient and are often collected inaccurately.

Nonproteinuric women may develop proteinuria during pregnancy due to hyperfiltration. Timed protein excretion of up to 300 mg/day or urine PCR of up to 30 mg/mmol can be observed in normal pregnancy.

Referral to a nephrologist

All women of child-bearing age, who have reduced GFR or albuminuria/proteinuria, require further investigation and usually warrant referral to a nephrologist, particularly if pregnancy is being contemplated. Additional investigations may include screening tests for autoimmune disease, renal imaging with ultrasound to identify anatomical abnormalities or cortical scarring, nuclear scans to assess for reflux nephropathy, and perhaps renal biopsy if no immediate cause of CKD is evident. Renal biopsy can be a key investigation and is best performed prior to pregnancy, although it can be safely performed in early pregnancy.

Management of CKD prepregnancy

The main aspects of prepregnancy management of women with CKD involve:

1. Diagnosis and treatment (if required) of underlying CKD and associated abnormalities particularly hypertension. This is best done before pregnancy to optimize the patient's condition and chances of successful pregnancy outcome.
2. Assessment of severity of CKD as measured by eGFR, urine protein excretion, biochemical abnormalities including acidosis, hyperkalemia and hyperphosphatemia, anemia, and hyperparathyroidism. This will guide counseling of the patient regarding fertility, pregnancy outcomes, and risks.
3. Medication review to enable use of pregnancy-safe drugs. The key drugs are angiotensin-converting enzyme (ACE) inhibitors and angiotensin II receptor blockers, which are widely utilized to delay progression of CKD, minimizing proteinuria and treating hypertension, particularly in diabetic nephropathy. It is currently

recommended that these drugs be ceased in pregnancy, as exposure in the second and third trimester is associated with growth restriction, oligohydramnios, renal dysplasia, fetal renal failure and fetal death. However, ceasing these drugs in pregnancy may lead to loss of their antiproteinuric effect.

Other significant drugs include immunosuppressive medications, the safety of which is outlined in detail in reference 3.

Outcomes of pregnancy in CKD patients

Effect of CKD on pregnancy outcomes

Pregnant women with CKD of any form have a 5-fold higher risk of adverse maternal events and 2-8 fold higher risk of adverse fetal events. In general, the degree of increased risk is closely linked to the severity of renal impairment and proteinuria prepregnancy, and control of hypertension during pregnancy. Women with a minor reduction in eGFR, minimal proteinuria, and normal blood pressure have the best prognosis. Women with more advanced CKD will have worse outcomes and may require more intensive management in pregnancy, often with a multidisciplinary team of clinicians.

Pregnant women with stage 1–2 CKD have a lower risk of adverse events, although still not equivalent to that of pregnant women without CKD. There is a 2-fold increased risk of preeclampsia, and a reported increased risk of prematurity and lower birth rate. Women with stage 3–4 CKD have a much lower overall fertility rate and increased risks of early and late fetal loss. They have a 50–60% rate of preeclampsia, which often occurs earlier and can be more severe. The prematurity rate is over 60%. Pregnancy in women with stage 5 CKD (on dialysis) is extremely rare and high risk. However, recent reports suggest that the live birth rate can be over 70% with intensive medical management. In general, women with advanced CKD are best counseled to defer pregnancy until after renal transplantation.

Fetal adverse events are related to the degree of biochemical abnormality, particularly increased maternal urea concentrations. There are higher rates of growth restriction, polyhydramnios related to fetal polyuria, prematurity, and risk of miscarriage or fetal death. Pregnant women with CKD require close fetal monitoring and serial growth scans.

Effect of pregnancy on CKD

- *Renal function:* Women with CKD in pregnancy have an increased risk of transient or permanent worsening of renal function and proteinuria, development of new hypertension or worsening of existing hypertension, and preeclampsia. Renal function may decline transiently or permanently in pregnancy, particularly in stage 3–4 CKD where 30–50% of women will have permanent nephron loss and decline in GFR. Failure of the GFR to increase physiologically in early pregnancy is an unfavorable prognostic feature and suggests inability of renal compensation. Rarely, renal function declines to the point where renal replacement therapy in pregnancy is required. Women with minimal renal impairment and well-controlled hypertension usually have no long-term adverse effect with pregnancy.
- *Proteinuria:* Existing proteinuria may worsen during pregnancy, occasionally reaching nephrotic degrees of protein excretion (>3 g/day). This may not always represent

preeclampsia or worsening renal disease. Women with severe nephrotic syndrome (urine protein excretion >6–10 g/day and severe hypoalbuminemia <12 g/L) should be considered for thromboprophylaxis, due to the increased thrombosis risk from urinary loss of anticoagulant proteins.

- *Hypertension:* Ideally, hypertension should be well controlled on pregnancy-safe medication prior to conception. Hypertension in women with CKD is extremely common and may be difficult to control. Severe hypertension will accelerate the decline in renal function. Hypertension in CKD pregnancies is difficult to differentiate from preeclampsia, as many of the parameters used for diagnosing preeclampsia (blood pressure, renal function, proteinuria, serum urate) may already be abnormal. Prophylaxis with low-dose aspirin should commence as early as possible and may reduce the risk of preeclampsia by 17%.

Summary

Women with CKD detected prior to pregnancy should be thoroughly investigated, and may require referral to a nephrologist. The degree of renal impairment and proteinuria, and the presence and control of hypertension, are the key factors determining the outcome of pregnancy. Women with minor (stage 1–2) CKD are at increased risk of adverse events but generally have favorable outcomes. Women with Stage 3–4 CKD must be counseled regarding the need for optimizing medical management prepregnancy, the need for close monitoring during pregnancy, and the heightened risks to both mother and baby.

References

1. Johnson DW *et al.* Chronic kidney disease and measurement of albuminuria or proteinuria: a position statement. Australasian Proteinuria Consensus Working Group. *Med J Aust* 2012; **197** (4): 224–5.

2. Kidney Health Australia Website http://www.kidney.org.au/; Detecting CKD.

3. Brahman K and Lightstone L. Pre-pregnancy counselling for women with chronic kidney disease. *J Nephrol* 2012; **25**(05): 450–9.

Further reading

Nevis IF *et al.* Pregnancy outcomes in women with chronic kidney disease: a systematic review. *Clin J Am Soc Nephrol* 2011; **6**(11): 2587–98.

Williams D and Davison J. Chronic kidney disease in pregnancy. *BMJ* 2008; **336**(7637): 211–15.

A male with oligozoospermia and muscle weakness subsequently diagnosed with myotonic dystrophy

Inge Liebaers and Willem Verpoest

Clinical fertility history

A young couple presented at the outpatient clinic for reproductive medicine. The woman was 32 years old, and her male partner 35 years old. Both were healthy. She had a 5-year-old healthy girl easily conceived with her previous partner, and he had a 10-year-old healthy boy from his first wife; the boy was born during the first year of their relationship and the couple separated when their child was 2 years old. The couple now had a desire to have children and despite regular intercourse for one year no pregnancy occurred. Developmental milestones of both partners, including pubertal development, had been normal. The woman resumed regular menstruation after having stopped the contraceptive pill.

General medical, family, and social history

The female partner had no relevant medical history. She was a highschool teacher, she played tennis, and her family history was unremarkable. The male partner had no medical complaints except for some daytime sleepiness and general fatigue, which limited his jogging activity. He worked as a journalist. His parents were reported to be in good health. His brother had three healthy children. His only sister had had a baby who had died perinatally; the baby was floppy and did not show spontaneous respiration at birth and despite adequate care the child did not survive. Diagnostic investigations were still ongoing at the time the couple presented.

Findings

Physical examination including gynecological and urogenital examination of both partners was normal, although the man was noted to have a sad, haggard facial expression and a slight ptosis of the upper eyelids. Nasal speech and frontal baldness were also noted.

Fertility investigations

The basic fertility investigations in the woman revealed normal serum gonadotropin (FSH, LH) and estrogen concentrations and a 46,XX karyotype. In the man FSH, LH, and testosterone concentrations were within the normal range. His karyotype was 46,XY. Sperm analysis revealed oligozoospermia with a sperm count below 5 million/mL.

Other clinical investigations

Further clinical examination of the male partner by a neurologist because of the fatigue, the eyelid ptosis, the nasal speech, the oligozoospermia, and the family history – namely his sister losing a floppy infant perinatally and his father presenting with cataract – revealed muscular weakness, percussion, and grip myotonia. The clinical diagnosis of myotonic dystrophy was suggested. A blood test looking for a CTG expansion in the untranslated 3′ region of the *DMPK1* gene on chromosome 19q13.3 was requested and showed the presence of 300 CTG repeats [1].

Diagnosis
The male partner had the adult form of myotonic dystrophy or Steinert disease [2, 3, 4].

Action plan
The couple was referred to a medical geneticist to be counseled on the possible symptoms of myotonic dystrophy as a multiorgan disorder as well as on the 50% risk of transmitting the condition in a more severe form to the offspring and discussing the possibilities for avoiding transmission. Taking into account the low sperm count on the one hand and the 50% risk of transmitting the disease, in vitro fertilization (IVF) by intracytoplasmic sperm injection (ICSI) and preimplantation genetic diagnosis (PGD) were proposed [5, 6].

Outcome
In the first treatment cycle eight cumulus–oocyte complexes (COCs) were retrieved and injected. Five oocytes were fertilized and four developed to the eight-cell stage. One embryo was unaffected and was transferred, but no pregnancy occurred. In the next treatment cycle again one unaffected embryo was transferred, resulting in a pregnancy followed by the birth of a healthy baby. A yearly multidisciplinary follow-up of the male partner was proposed.

General remarks
Faced with an infertile couple, it is important to take a careful personal and family history and to perform a general physical examination. Male infertility due to decreasing sperm quality is not uncommon in myotonic dystrophy. Myotonic dystrophy type 1 is, with a frequency of 1/5000 to 1/10 000, the most common muscular dystrophy in adults. Because it is an autosomal dominant condition, the recurrence risk is 50%. Moreover, the severity of the disease increases in successive generations due to the increase of the trinucleotide expansion being more pronounced in the female meiosis and most probably explaining the congenital form of the condition in his sister's baby. A loose correlation exists between the size of the expansion measured by the number of CTG repeats and the clinical expression, which can be mild (between 50 and 100–150 repeats), juvenile and adult-onset or classic (150 to 1000 repeats), and congenital (over 1000 repeats). Unaffected people have between 5 and 37 stable repeats while others have between 38 and 50 unstable repeats and are therefore termed premutation carriers by some. Due to the molecular complexity of the condition described in short as a splicopathy causing dysfunction of downstream effector genes, it is also a multisystem disorder characterized by cataract, endocrine problems, and cardiac conduction defects and cognitive problems. Especially women affected by mild or classic myotonic dystrophy should have a cardiac evaluation before infertility treatment and pregnancy and general anesthesia should be avoided [1, 2, 3, 4]. The rather complex genetic counseling should be offered not only to the couple but also to other at-risk members of the family [7].

References

1. Kamsteeg EJ, Kress W, Catalli C, Hertz JM, Witsch-Baumgartner M, Buckley MF, van Engelen BG, Schwartz M, Scheffer H. Best practice guidelines and recommendations on the molecular diagnosis of myotonic dystrophy types 1 and 2. *Eur J Hum Genet* 2012; **20**(12): 1203–8.

2. Udd B, Krahe R. The myotonic dystrophies: molecular, clinical, and therapeutic challenges.*Lancet Neurol* 2012; **11**(10): 891–905.

3. Romeo V. Myotonic dystrophy type 1 or Steinert's disease. [Review]. *Adv Exp Med Biol* 2012; **724**: 239–57.

4. Kim WB, Jeong JY, Doo SW, Yang WJ, Song YS, Lee SR, Park JW, Kim DW. Myotonic dystrophy type 1 presenting as male infertility.*Korean J Urol* 2012; **53**(2): 134–6.

5. Verpoest W, De Rademaeker M, Sermon K, De Rycke M, Seneca S, Papanikolaou E, Spits C, Van Landuyt L, Van der Elst J, Haentjens P, Devroey P, Liebaers I. Real and expected delivery rates of patients with myotonic dystrophy undergoing intracytoplasmic sperm injection and preimplantation genetic diagnosis. *Hum Reprod* 2008; **23**(7): 1654–60.

6. De Rademaeker M, Verpoest W, De Rycke M, Seneca S, Sermon K, Desmyttere S, Bonduelle M, Van der Elst J, Devroey P, Liebaers I.Preimplantation genetic diagnosis for myotonic dystrophy type 1: upon request to child.*Eur J Hum Genet* 2009; **17**(11): 1403–10.

7. Bird TD. Myotonic Dystrophy Type 1. *GeneReviews [Internet]* 2013; Bookshelf ID: NBK1165; http://www.ncbi.nlm.nih.gov/books/NBK1165/.

Never say never to a Klinefelter patient

Inge Liebaers and Herman Tournaye

Clinical fertility history

A young couple was referred to the Center for Medical Genetics for investigation following the occurrence of an unexpected pregnancy. The woman was 26 years old and her developmental milestones and pubertal development were normal. She had regular menses. She had obtained a university degree and was responsible for clinical trials in a pharmaceutical company. Her male partner was also 26 years old, was well, and worked as sales manager at the same pharmaceutical company as his wife. Before their marriage, he had informed his future partner that he was not able to have children because when he was a child the diagnosis of Klinfelter syndrome had been established, following investigation of speech delay and some learning difficulties. Because of the unexpected pregnancy, he was convinced that she had been unfaithful to him and asked for paternity testing. A spontaneous miscarriage occurred, but paternity testing was possible through DNA fingerprinting and confirmed that the male partner was indeed the genetic father. Two years later they presented at the fertility clinic asking for help to conceive again.

General medical, family, and social history

The general medical history of the couple did not reveal any particular or relevant problem. Each partner had healthy parents and a healthy sibling with two healthy children. The man mentioned that with educational support he had been able to complete high school and he obtained a bachelor degree. He did not report any behavioral problems.

Examination findings

The woman had a completely normal physical and gynecological examination. The male partner was tall with a degree of truncal obesity and slight gynecomastia. His testes were small and his beard growth was shallow.

Fertility investigations

The woman reported regular menstrual periods and early follicular phase FSH and estrogen levels were normal. Her karyotype was 46,XX. The man had increased FSH levels, a high LH concentration, and a low–normal testosterone concentration. His karyotype was 47,XXY. Sperm analysis showed azoospermia in two serial samples.

Other clinical investigations

No further investigations were planned for either partner.

Diagnosis

A clearcut diagnosis of nonmosaic 47,XXY, Klinefelter syndrome was confirmed in the man. The azoospermia was the cause of the infertility – but what about the one pregnancy?

Action plan

A diagnostic testes biopsy was proposed in order to find out whether some spermatogenic activity was still present. If it was not, artificial insemination of the wife with donor sperm could be offered. If spermatogenic activity and spermatozoa were found, in vitro fertilization(IVF) with intracytoplasmic sperm injection (ICSI) could be proposed, with the explanation that in case of pregnancy, although the risk for aneuploidy in the fetus may slightly be increased, most of the recorded children born so far with ICSI without preimplantation genetic diagnosis (PGD) had a "normal" karyotype. In fact a rate of only 1/100 children with a 47,XXY karyotype has been reported [1, 2]. Nevertheless, the possibility of PGD was discussed [1, 2]

Outcome

Since spermatozoa were found in the testes, the couple opted for IVF with ICSI and PGD. In two consecutive cycles, ten cumulus–oocyte complexes (COCs) could be retrieved and ten oocytes were injected with one spermatozoon, seven of these oocytes were fertilized and five embryos developed until the 8-cell stage. In the first cycle three embryos were aneuploid for one of the tested chromosomes 13, 16, 18, 21, 22, X, and Y and two were euploid. One embryo was transferred at the blastocyst stage but no pregnancy occurred. The remaining embryo could not be frozen because of bad morphological quality. In the second cycle, two euploid embryos were transferred but again no pregnancy occurred. The couple asked for a third treatment cycle without PGD; in case of pregnancy, they had the intention to undergo an amniocentesis, but again no pregnancy could be established. They then asked for artificial insemination with donor sperm and were counseled and prepared for it. After three inseminations, the wife was pregnant and a healthy baby was born.

General remarks

Klinefelter syndrome, although seemingly well known, has an extremely variable and sometimes confusing clinical presentation [3, 4]. According to one study, up to 75% of Klinefelter patients remain undiagnosed. Once azoospermia has been diagnosed, up to 11% of these men have a 47,XXY karyotype, which is nonmosaic in 80–90% of the cases [2]. The classic signs of adult 47,XXY patients are small testes due to progressive fibrosis and hyalinization of the seminiferous tubules, high FSH and LH levels, variable testosterone levels from normal to low but most of the time a high LH/testosterone ratio, and a tall stature. In a clinical study of 166 boys and adults with Klinefelter syndrome, cryptorchidism was observed in 14% of the patients and gynecomastia in 44%, and speech therapy or educational support had been necessary in 36% [5]. Klinefelter patients are also prone to other medical problems such as tumors especially the rare mediastinal germ cell tumors, vascular disease, and endocrine disease such as diabetes mellitus and metabolic syndrome [6]. Although patients are usually azoospermic, in up to 8% of nonmosaic patients spermatozoa can be found in the ejaculate, which may explain the pregnancy in our couple [2]. The message to an azoospermic Klinefelter patient is, therefore, not that he will never become a father but that these chances are very low. Similarly to testicular sperm recovery rates in non-Klinefelter azoospermic patients with primary testicular failure, focal spermatogenesis is observed in about 50% of cases, a figure similar to that in nonadult adolescent Klinefelter boys [7, 8]. With extraction of spermatozoa from the testicular tissue and use of ICSI, these patients may have a chance to father their own child, usually presenting with a normal karyotype [1, 2] Two hypotheses have been proposed to explain spermatogenesis leading to the production of "normal" as well as abnormal spermatozoa. One is based on the assumption that XXY-spermatogonia can complete meiosis and produce X and Y spermatozoa as well as XX and XY spermatozoa. The other hypothesis assumes that, in the testes, patches of XY spermatogonia occur but the testicular environment is conducive to meiotic errors resulting an increased number of XX, YY, and XY spermatozoa next to X and Y spermatozoa. Evidence supporting both hypotheses exists but no final conclusion can be drawn at present [9]. Offering testicular tissue banking to young Klinefelter patients to overcome the reported stem cell depletion later in life and eventually preserve fertility should be considered experimental at this time, as many unresolved questions remain [8]. Cryopreservation of sperm if they are found in the ejaculate may be an effective option in some men [10]. Finally, testosterone substitution is widely used to treat symptoms of hypogonadism but should be individualized [11].

References

1. Staessen C, Tournaye H, Van Assche E, Michiels A, Van Landuyt L, Devroey P, Liebaers I, Van Steirteghem A. PGD in 47,XXY Klinefelter's syndrome patients. [Review]. *Hum Reprod Update* 2003; **9**(4): 319–30.

2. Fullerton G, Hamilton M, Maheshwari A Should non-mosaic Klinefelter syndrome men be labelled as infertile in 2009? *Hum Reprod.* 2010; **25**(3): 588–97.

3. Sigman M.Klinefelter syndrome: how, what, and why? *Fertil Steril* 2012; **98**(2): 251–2.

4. Juul A, Aksglaede L, Bay K, Grigor KM, Skakkebaek NE. Klinefelter syndrome: the forgotten syndrome: basic and clinical questions posed to an international group of scientists. *Acta Paediatr* 2011; **100**(6): 791–2.

5. Aksglaede L, Skakkebaek NE, Almstrup K, Juul A. Clinical and biological parameters in 166 boys, adolescents and adults with nonmosaic Klinefelter syndrome: a Copenhagen experience. *Acta Paediatr* 2011; **100**(6): 793–806.

6. Sokol RZ. It's not all about the testes: medical issues in Klinefelter patients. *Fertil Steril* 2012; **98**(2): 261–5.

7. Tournaye H, Staessen C, Liebaers I, Van Assche E, Devroey P, Bonduelle M *et al.* Testicular sperm recovery in nine 47,XXY Klinefelter patients. *Hum Reprod* 1996; **11**: 1650–3.

8. Gies I, De Schepper J, Goossens E, Van Saen D, Pennings G, Tournaye H. Spermatogonial stem cell preservation in boys with Klinefelter syndrome: to bank or not to bank, that's the question. *Fertil Steril* 2012; **98**(2): 284–9.

9. Maiburg M, Repping S, Giltay J. The genetic origin of Klinefelter syndrome and its effect on spermatogenesis. *Fertil Steril* 2012; **98**(2): 253–60.

10. Oates RD. The natural history of endocrine function and spermatogenesis in Klinefelter syndrome: what the data show. *Fertil Steril* 2012; **98**(2): 266–73.

11 Wikström AM, Dunkel L. Klinefelter syndrome. *Best Pract Res Clin Endocrinol Metab* 2011; **25**(2): 239–50.

A man with retrograde ejaculation

S. Alberto Dávila Garza and Pasquale Patrizio

Clinical fertility history

Mrs. S.K. (33 years) and Mr. K.K. (32 years) are an American couple who presented with infertility after one year of unprotected intercourse. Mr. K.K. was diagnosed with diabetes mellitus type 1 when he was 16 years old. He remained under treatment with his primary care physician and, when referred, reported good control. Two years previously he had developed erectile dysfunction, which was treated with 5-phosphodiesterase inhibitors. A good response was reported but he noticed a decrease in the ejaculate volume. The couple had not previously been investigated for infertility.

General medical, family, and social history

Mrs. S.K. presented as a healthy woman, nonsmoker, G1 P1, with an unremarkable medical and surgical history. She reported irregular cycles every 32 to 42 days, of 5 days duration and with normal menstrual flow. No dysmenorrhea was described. Her first pregnancy was uneventful, apart from requiring a cesarean section for failure to progress during labor.

Mr. K.K. presented otherwise as a healthy nonsmoker. He maintained normal glucose levels under stable insulin therapy. He was also taking an angiotensin-converting enzyme (ACE) inhibitor for kidney protection.

Physical examination

Mrs. S.K. weighed 59 kg with a body mass index of 22.0 kg/m². Mr. K.K. weighed 68 kg with a body mass index of 22.0 kg/m². General examination was unremarkable in both. Female pelvic examination was unremarkable, and male genital examination revealed normal external genitalia with the vas deferens present on both sides.

Fertility investigations

Mrs. S.K had normal cycle day 3 FSH, LH, and estradiol levels, and a mid-luteal progesterone consistent with ovulation. The antimüllerian hormone (AMH) level was 2.24 ng/mL. Infection and further endocrine screening were normal. An ultrasound scan showed a normal anteverted uterus, normal ovaries, and a combined antral follicle count of 8. Hysterosalpingography (HSG) showed bilateral tubal patency.

Mr. K.K.'s semen analysis revealed aspermia. Repeat semen analysis using a retrograde ejaculation protocol indicated aspermia and a urine pH of 6.0. However, after centrifugation a volume of 0.5 mL of sperm cells was isolated with a concentration was 13.6 million/mL, total sperm motility 17%, sperm morphology 32% abnormal forms. Hepatitis B serology and hepatitis C serology were negative.

Other clinical investigations

Due to Mrs. S.K.'s ovulatory dysfunction, investigations for suspected polycystic ovary syndrome were performed, showing normal glucose, hemoglobin A1$_c$ and serum insulin with total and free testosterone also in the normal range.

Diagnosis

One year of secondary infertility likely related to retrograde ejaculation and mild ovulatory dysfunction.

Treatment

The couple was advised to undergo ovulation induction and intrauterine insemination in the first instance. Three cycles of ovulation induction were performed using recombinant follicle-stimulating hormone (rFSH) 75 IU starting on the third day of the menstrual cycle. Ultrasound monitoring was done until the dominant follicle(s) reached ≥18 mm diameter.

Yale retrograde ejaculation protocol sample collection

The following protocol was used.

- 1 tablet of sodium bicarbonate dissolved in a half glass of water prior to the evening meal.
- Avoid acid foods the night before (vinegar, salad dressing, wine, tomatoes, etc.).
- After the evening meal, 2 tablets of sodium bicarbonate dissolved in water.

On the morning of the sample collection:

- 2 tablets of sodium bicarbonate dissolved in water.
- Urinate 30 minutes prior to collecting the sample (to avoid excessively amount of urine at sample collection time).
- Obtain the sample by masturbation and collect any amount of seminal fluid that might be discharged in a sterile container.
- Following this, collect the first urine after ejaculation in a sterile cup.
- 2 tablets of a sympathomimetic agent (such as pseudoephedrine) orally

The sample was analyzed and processed immediately.

Reproductive outcome

Following intrauterine insemination (IUI) with the sperm thus obtained, one biochemical pregnancy was achieved in the first cycle, and a clinical pregnancy was obtained after the third attempt. A single intrauterine pregnancy was observed with a positive fetal heartbeat.

General remarks

Retrograde ejaculation is an uncommon cause of male infertility, being reported in less than 2% of the infertile population [1]. The presence of aspermia (absence of semen) or very low semen volume is highly suspicious of this clinical entity [2]. To understand the mechanism, knowledge of the normal ejaculation process is required. Ejaculation is a sympathetic neuro-complex mechanism that is triggered as a result of mechanical stimulation of the penis [3].

Antegrade propulsion results from the tightening of the closed bladder neck, relaxation of the external sphincter, and contraction of the bulbocavernosus muscle [4]. These processes require the synchrony of three different mechanisms:

1. Closure of the bladder neck, controlled by the ventral roots of T12 to L3 spinal nerves.
2. Seminal emission, which involves the movement of semen into the posterior urethra prior to ejaculation controlled by T12–L3.
3. Ejaculation or expulsion, which is the passage of semen through the urethra.

Retrograde ejaculation involves a partial or total failure of this mechanism [5] due to either structural or functional disruption of the process [2]. The most common causes described include congenital abnormalities, spinal trauma, retroperitoneal lymph node resection (i.e., testicular cancer), diabetes mellitus, or idiopathic multiple sclerosis.

The treatment of this condition can be either medical or surgical correction to restore antegrade ejaculation. Medical treatment aims at increasing the tone of the bladder neck by either stimulating sympathetic activity or blocking parasympathetic stimulation. The approach used in the fertility clinic aims to improve the normally adverse environment in the bladder to be able to recover sufficient sperm with minimal deleterious impact on quality, before processing them to perform assisted reproduction [3].

Comments

Long-term side effects of diabetes mellitus include peripheral neuropathy; even with good control this may not be avoided. Erectile dysfunction and retrograde ejaculation account for around 13% of cases of male infertility [6]. The approach used was aimed at preparing the bladder to avoid the detrimental effect of the acid pH and osmolarity of the urine on sperm [5]. Sympathomimetic agents (such as pseudoephedrine) may result in antegrade ejaculation in up to 28% of cases. A pregnancy rate per cycle using intrauterine insemination of 15% has been described in a recent meta-analysis [3]. Other assisted reproductive technologies such as in vitro fertilization with or without testicular sperm recovery can be used, but management needs to be tailored individually and according to the current partner's fertility status.

References

1. Yavetz H, Yogev L, Hauser R, Lessing J, Paz G, Hommanai ZT. Retrograde ejaculation. *Hum Reprod Update* 1994; **9**: 381–6.

2. Jarvi K, Roberts M. Steps in the investigation and management of low volume semen in the infertile men. *Can Urol Assoc J* 2009; **3**(6): 479–85.

3. Jefferys A, Wardle P, Siassakos D. The management of retrograde ejaculation: a systematic review and update. *Fert Steril* 2012; **97**(2): 306–12.

4. Steele G, Richie J. Retroperitoneal lymph node dissection in testicular germ cell tumors. *UpToDate*, March 21, 2012.

5. Aust T *et al*. Development and in vitro testing of a new method of urine preparation for retrograde ejaculation: The Liverpool solution. *Fert Steril* 2008; **89**(4): 885–91.

6. Kamischke A, Nieschlag E. Mini-symposium: non surgical sperm recovery: Part II. Treatment of retrograde ejaculation and anejaculation. *Hum Reprod Update* 1999; **5**(5): 448–74.

Chapter 9

A patient with severe lupus

Erin Clark and William M. Hague

Clinical history

Mrs. A. was a 31-year-old housewife from the eastern suburbs of Adelaide, Australia, whose first pregnancy 5 years earlier while in Greece had been complicated by severe preeclampsia at 31 weeks gestation, delivering a growth-restricted infant, birth weight 900 g, who has a learning disability. A month after delivery, she had a pulmonary embolism and was treated with warfarin for 6 months. She had ongoing proteinuria (2 g/24 h) and on investigation was found to have normal blood count and renal function, ANA 1/640 homogeneous, double-stranded DNA antibody 32 U/L, complement levels were normal, cardiolipin antibody and lupus anticoagulant tities were negative. She refused renal biopsy and, after returning to Australia, had come off her medications a year previously, since when she had been trying to conceive with normal menses. At presentation she had a facial rash, her blood pressure was normal, and urinalysis showed 2+ protein and a trace of blood.

Case discussion

Mrs. A. had a history and clinical features which would fit with a diagnosis of systemic lupus erythematosus (SLE), possibly complicated by lupus nephritis. SLE is a multisystem auto-immune disease characterized by a relapsing and remitting course. It is more common in women than in men, with a peak onset during the childbearing stage (20–40 years). While SLE does not *per se* adversely affect fertility, adverse pregnancy outcomes are more commonly seen in affected women. They require the involvement of a multidisciplinary team with careful assessment and increased maternal and fetal surveillance during pregnancy.

There are a number of factors known to increase the risk of adverse pregnancy outcomes in women with SLE; conversely, for those women who do not have any of these risk factors, the likelihood of pregnancy problems appears comparable with that of the general population. These risk factors are:

- Active disease at conception or within 6 months prior
- Hypertension
- Renal disease (elevated creatinine, proteinuria ≥0.5 g/24 h)
- Anti-phospholipid antibodies (lupus anticoagulant, cardiolipin antibodies, beta-2 glycoprotein-1 antibodies)
- Anti-Ro (SSA) or anti-La (SSB) antibodies.

The following issues need to be considered:

1. What features of this patient's history should raise concerns with regard to both fertility treatment and pregnancy? What other complications of SLE should be assessed prior to fertility treatment/pregnancy?

2. What potential risks to both mother and baby need to be discussed?
3. For women with SLE presenting pre conception (or in early pregnancy), assessment of both functional organ damage and disease activity is required. What investigations would assist in making this assessment?
4. Are there any particular medication concerns?
5. After consideration of all issues, how should this woman be counseled?

Mrs. A.'s history was suggestive of renal lupus, but the degree of renal impairment and current disease activity was uncertain. Her story suggested the onset of SLE with lupus nephritis during pregnancy, which may well have been the cause of her severe, early-onset preeclampsia. While lupus nephritis and preeclampsia can be difficult to distinguish clinically, and proteinuria can persist for up to 6 months following severe preeclampsia, the presence of a moderate titer of double-stranded DNA (ds-DNA) antibody points to SLE. Renal biopsy, had it been performed, could have provided confirmation of renal lupus, classification of subtype, and a measure of severity. More recently, the presence of blood and protein on urinalysis points to renal involvement (possibly active disease, which is not excluded by the absence of hypertension) and warrants thorough assessment.

Additionally, she had been off medication for 12 months and had a facial rash, which again suggested active lupus. Other symptoms such as arthralgia, myalgia, fatigue, headaches, and mouth ulcers may have been present, and should be elicited on history. It is also important to ask about any history of cardiac and respiratory involvement, as well as symptoms such as reduced exercise tolerance, cough, and dyspnea. Pulmonary hypertension can occur in up to 14% of women with SLE, and is a contraindication to pregnancy due to the high rate of maternal mortality in affected women.

Mrs. A. had also suffered a postpartum pulmonary embolism, which increases her risk of subsequent thromboembolic events, particularly post partum, but also both in pregnancy and during fertility treatment if hormonal manipulation is required. She did not appear to have anti-phospholipid antibodies, which are present in up to 40% of women with SLE and increase the risk of both thromboembolic events (arterial and venous) and obstetric complications. However, she had not been tested for beta-2-glycoprotein-1 antibodies, a more specific risk marker for thrombosis in SLE. In addition, anti-phospholipid antibody titers can vary with time, so that repeat assay of both cardiolipin antibodies and lupus anticoagulant is worthwhile.

During the nine months of pregnancy, women with SLE have an increased risk of disease flares (40% nonpregnant vs. 60% of pregnant patients); these flares are generally mild and usually involve skin and joints. There is also an increased risk of flares during hormonal manipulation. Factors which increase the likelihood and severity of flares are a history of renal involvement and active disease in the 6 months prior to conception. The risk of flare in pregnancy is such that continuation of immunosuppressive agents, such as azathioprine or hydroxychloroquine, is considered essential, with minimal risk to the developing fetus. Flares in pregnancy can be treated with increased doses of steroids and the addition of other immunosuppressive drugs, such as cyclosporine (ciclosporin) or tacrolimus. There is a 30% chance of a renal flare during pregnancy; this risk is increased (50–60%) if there is active nephritis or partial remission at conception. While high-dose steroids can be used to treat lupus nephritis, severe episodes may require the use of cyclophosphamide or mycophenylate, both of which are contraindicated in the first trimester of pregnancy, although there may be a case to use these drugs later in pregnancy. Monoclonal antibody therapy (e.g., rituximab) may be considered in severe cases, although neonatal B-cell depletion has been reported occurring for up to six months from exposure.

Women with lupus have increased rates of preeclampsia, intrauterine growth restriction, fetal loss, and preterm delivery. Recent series have placed the live birth rate at 86–89%, with an incidence of preterm delivery of 31–44% and of preeclampsia occurring in up to 20%. Renal disease, even if quiescent, increases the risk of these complications; the likelihood is greater if features such as proteinuria or hypertension are present. The presence of anti-phospholipid antibodies in particular is associated with an increased rate of fetal loss.

Approximately 30% of women with SLE will have positive anti-Ro (SSA) and/or anti-La (SSB) on testing for extractable nuclear antigens (ENA). These antigens can cross the placenta, with an associated risk of neonatal lupus and congenital heart block (CHB) in the fetus; the rates are 5% and 2% respectively. Neonatal lupus commonly presents with a mild transient rash which requires no specific treatment. More rarely, it can be complicated by hemolytic anemia, thrombocytopenia, hepatitis, nephritis, aseptic meningitis, and myelopathy. CHB is generally not detected until after 18 weeks gestation. Once present, it is generally irreversible and is associated with a high rate of morbidity and mortality (20–30% neonatal mortality). Sixty percent of surviving children will require a pacemaker by the age of 12 years. The risk of both neonatal lupus and CHB increases with an affected sibling (17–25%), and may be up to 50% if there are two affected siblings; in general, these two complications do not coexist. There is currently no specific treatment available to prevent or treat fetal heart block associated with maternal SSA/SSB antibody. Mrs. A.'s ENA titers and further information regarding her child's neonatal history will enable more specific counseling regarding the risk in this area.

Baseline investigations should include complete blood picture, electrolytes, urea and creatinine, liver function tests, and inflammatory markers. Serological testing for antinuclear antibodies (ANA), ENA, ds-DNA antibody, complement components, and anti-phospholipid antibodies, as well as screening for lupus anticoagulant, should also be performed. It may also be appropriate to test for genetic thrombophilia (factor V Leiden, prothrombin gene mutation, antithrombin, protein C and protein S deficiencies), if these had not been checked at the time of her pulmonary embolism, and particularly if there is any close family history of thromboembolic disease. Both a spun urine looking for an active sediment (indicating active nephritis), and a quantitative 24-hour urine protein estimation should be obtained. Renal ultrasound and referral to a nephrologist for consideration of renal biopsy is indicated if significant proteinuria (>1 g/24 h) is present or the spun urine indicates nephritis. It may also be appropriate to investigate her cardiac/respiratory status with electrocardiography (ECG), echocardiography, and pulmonary function tests.

Once Mrs. A.'s SLE has been fully assessed and a treatment plan made, discussion between the fertility clinic and any treating physicians (nephrologist/rheumatologist/hematologist/obstetric physician) should be ongoing, particularly in the area of medication use and timing of fertility treatment. There are many immunosuppressive agents which can be safely continued in pregnancy, and, if relevant, Mrs. A. should be advised to remain on them throughout fertility treatment and pregnancy. Alternatively, she may require agents such as mycophenolate or cyclophosphamide, which are known to be teratogenic and which require some months' washout prior to conception. Premature ovarian failure is more common in women treated with cyclophosphamide over the age of 32 years, and its occurrence is directly proportional to the cumulative lifetime dose. Mrs. A.'s previous medication history should be obtained from Greece, and if appropriate, fertility-sparing treatment may need to be explored.

In women with a history of early-onset preeclampsia, antenatal use of low-dose aspirin (75–150 mg daily) has been shown to reduce the risk of recurrence by 17%. Both aspirin and calcium supplementation are indicated in Mrs. A., and should be started from early in pregnancy (see Chapter 2 on hypertension).

In women with a history of thromboembolism, low-molecular-weight heparin (LMWH) or warfarin is indicated for postnatal thromboprophylaxis, and should be administered for at least 6 weeks post delivery. Antenatal thromboprophylaxis in such women should be guided by the presence of anti-phospholipid antibodies; if they are present in moderate to high titers, antenatal LMWH should be considered. The dose (prophylactic or therapeutic) should be decided in consultation with her treating physicians. Antenatal thromboprophylaxis could also be considered if she should be found to carry a genetic thrombophilia in the absence of anti-phospholipid antibodies.

Serious consideration needs to be given to whether the risk of potentially fatal recurrent thromboembolism should contraindicate the use of ovulation induction agents, especially if IVF and associated superovulation treatment with its associated risk of severe ovarian hyperstimulation syndrome (OHSS) is being considered. A case–control register study from Norway has shown a 4-fold increase in risk of antenatal thromboembolism following assisted reproduction, with no reference to previous history or treatment. Almost half of these patients had suffered severe OHSS, in which thromboprophylaxis is considered a standard precaution. The risk for thromboembolic disease in IVF pregnancies has been estimated to be twice that of non-IVF pregnancies after controlling for age, parity, and smoking, while the incidence of thromboembolism is 0.04 to 0.2% in IVF cycles without OHSS and 4% in cycles complicated by OHSS. There are no good data on the efficacy and risks of thromboprophylaxis in assisted reproduction.

Mrs. A.'s story has features which suggest both renal lupus and active disease. These two things increase the risk of both significant disease flares in pregnancy and poor pregnancy outcomes. Deferring fertility treatment until her medical condition has been fully assessed, appropriate treatment has been instituted, and her SLE having been in complete remission for at least 6 months will significantly reduce the likelihood of disease flares and improve pregnancy outcomes. Further discussion regarding her specific risks during fertility treatment and pregnancy should occur after she has been fully assessed and stabilized on treatment. In addition, a formal plan for a multidisciplinary approach to monitoring her condition throughout fertility treatment and pregnancy should be put in place, preferably prior to starting. This should also include the involvement of obstetric services for any required fetal surveillance.

Further reading

Bramham K, Soh MC and, Nelson-Piercy C. Pregnancy and renal outcomes in lupus nephritis: an update and guide to management. *Lupus* 2011; 21: 1271–83.

Jacobsen AF, Skjeldestad FE and, Sandse PM. Incidence and risk patterns of venous thromboembolism in pregnancy and puerperium – a register-based case-control study. *American Journal of Obstetrics and Gynecology* 2008; **198** (2): 233.e1–7.

Kwok L-K, Tam L-S, Zhu T, Leung YY and, Li E. Predictors of maternal and fetal outcomes in pregnancies of patients with systemic lupus erythematosus. *Lupus* 2011; **20**: 829–36.

MacKillop LH, Germaine SJ, Nelson-Piercy C. Pregnancy Plus: Systemic lupus erythematosus. *BMJ* 2007; **335**: 933–6.

Nelson-Piercy C. Connective-tissue disease. In: Nelson-Piercy C. (ed.) *Handbook of Obstetric Medicine*, 4th edn. London: Informa Healthcare ; 2010; 129–50.

Weinerman R, Grifo J. Consequences of superovulation and ART procedures. *Seminars in Reproductive Medicine* 2012; **30** (2):77–83.

Chapter 10

One partner is a carrier of thalassemia, one a carrier of sickle cell anemia

Human M. Fatemi

Clinical fertility history

A 32-year-old nulligravida patient of Congolese origin with a 2-year history of primary infertility presented for an IVF treatment after failure to conceive with six cycles of ovulation induction and intrauterine insemination. The patient had been previously diagnosed with an intramural fibroid of 4 cm which did not impinge on the endometrial cavity. A hysterosalpingogram performed 6 months prior to the visit had demonstrated bilateral patent tubes and a normal shape of the uterine cavity

General medical, family, and social history

The patient had no previous medical history of note and no previous family history of sickle cell anemia. Her husband, a white man of Italian origin had also no known previous medical history of note and no family history of thalassemia. The couple were nonsmokers and nondrinkers.

Examination findings

The patient had a BMI of 22 kg/m^2 and general physical examination was completely normal. On bimanual examination a large fibroid was confirmed. No other abnormalities were evident.

Fertility investigations

On day 3 of the cycle, the patient had a normal endocrine profile with an FSH level of 4.5 IU/L, LH of 3.2 IU/L, progesterone of 0.2 ng/mL, and an estradiol of 320 pmol/L. On transvaginal ultrasound, her ovaries were visible and antral follicle counts (AFC) of 7 on the right and 5 on the left ovary were observed. A posterior intramural fibroid of 4 cm in diameter was visualized without having any compression on the uterine cavity. No other abnormalities of her internal genitalia were detected.

A diagnostic hysteroscopy was performed and confirmed the absence of any compression into the cavity. Her partner's semen analysis parameters were within the normal range.

Other clinical investigations

A karyotype of both partners was done which was completely normal. Moreover, her complete blood count (CBC) levels were within the normal range.

Diagnosis

Primary idiopathic infertility was diagnosed, since there is limited scientific evidence that the fibroid would be the cause of the infertility.

Action plan

The patient and her partner were advised to start IVF treatment.

A first rec-FSH/GnRH antagonist treatment with a good response: nine cumulus–oocyte complexes were retrieved and one good-quality blastocyst was transferred. However, the pregnancy test after 2 weeks was negative. After discussing the case in detail with both partners, it was decided to perform a laparoscopic myomectomy.

The operation was done without any complications. After 4 months, the patient started a new IVF cycle using the same stimulation protocol.

Outcome

The patient conceived and at 7 weeks a singleton intrauterine pregnancy was confirmed by ultrasound. The pregnancy was uneventful. During labor at term, the patient underwent cesarean section for fetal distress. After the delivery, the baby was transferred to the intensive care unit suffering from the effects of hypoxia. A clinically significant anemia was diagnosed and found to derive from the co-inheritance of a β-thalassemia mutation from the father and a mutation that results in production of a mutant β-globin chain from the mother (hemoglobin S, HbS).

This combination is clinically similar to that in a patient with β-thalassemia major, which is a clinically severe thalassemia. The baby was treated appropriately and was discharged after 3 weeks of intensive care unit treatment.

Discussion

The thalassemia syndromes and related hemoglobinopathies are the commonest group of monogenic disorders worldwide [1]. β-Thalassemia is an autosomal recessive disorder caused by mutations in the β-globin gene located on chromosome 11. People who inherit two β-thalassemia mutations usually have β-thalassemia major, a severe dyserythropoietic anemia requiring life-long treatment with blood transfusions to maintain satisfactory levels of hemoglobin and iron-chelation therapy to combat the tendency to iron overload.

Whereas the thalassemias are caused by gene mutations resulting in decreased production of α- or β-globin chains, the sickle cell disorders are hemoglobinopathies caused by mutations in the β-globin gene resulting in the production of a structurally abnormal β-globin chain. This abnormal hemoglobin, HbS, forms a gel polymer under conditions of low oxygen tension. Collectively, the polymerized Hb molecules force the red cell into a sickle shape, and such a cell may become trapped in small blood vessels, causing a wide variety of clinically severe complications and increased mortality in affected individuals. Homozygotes are characterized by lifelong hemolytic anemia with increased morbidity and mortality associated with a variety of complications related to the deleterious effects of vaso-occlusive episodes and increased propensity to infection.

Since those disorders are recessive, many patients are asymptomatic and the CBC will show mild or no anemia.

In countries with an ethnic population at an increased risk for thalassemia or sickle cell disorders, genetic counseling, ideally in the preconception period should be advised.

Given the autosomal recessive nature of thalassemia and sickle cell disorders, the identification of any individual as a carrier indicates that the mutation is segregating in the family. Carriers need to be informed that their siblings, their children, and other family members are at increased risk of being carriers and should discuss the matter with their health care providers.

In this specific case, however, the parents were of different ethnic origins: southern European (Italian) and black African (Congo), without any familial history of known hemoglobinopathies.

Moreover, each parent was the carrier of a different mutation; β-thalassemia and heterozygous sickle hemoglobinopathy. One would think given the different forms of hemoglobinopathy mutations (thalassemia and sickle cell) that no disease would occur. However, clinically significant disease can occur from the co-inheritance of a β-thalassemia mutation from one parent and a HbS mutation that results in production of a mutant globin chain from the other parent.

If both partners are found to be carriers of hemoglobin mutations (i.e., any combination of thalassemias and Hb variants), they should be referred for genetic counseling, ideally in the preconception period, or as early as possible in the pregnancy. Additional molecular studies may be required to clarify the risk to the fetus. The main approach for controlling severe genetic diseases remains prevention, and preimplantation genetic diagnosis represents an alternative procedure [2] in the context of prenatal diagnostic services, heralded as a means of avoiding the trauma and ethical dilemma of terminating affected pregnancies.

References

1. Weatherall DJ. Single gene disorders or complex traits: lessons from thalassaemia and other monogenic diseases. *Br Med J* 2000; **321**: 1117–20.

2. Traeger-Synodinos J, Vrettou C, Palmer G *et al.* An evaluation of PGD in clinical genetic services through 3 years application for prevention of β-thalassaemia major and sickle cell thalassaemia *Mol Hum Reprod* 2003; **9**(5): 301–7.

A patient with Kallmann syndrome

Dimitra Kyrou

Clinical fertility history

A 28-year-old nulliparous woman, married for 3 years, was referred to our clinic for investigation due to primary infertility. Her partner had normal sperm quality parameters according to World Health Organization standards. The patient had embarked on one cycle of intrauterine insemination (IUI) 6 months previously. However, this was cancelled when no follicular response to human menopausal gonadotropin (hMG) was observed after 15 days of ovarian stimulation.

General medical history

The patient presented at the age of 17 years with a history of primary amenorrhea and anosmia. She demonstrated very low serum levels of FSH (2.12 IU/L), LH (0.40 IU/L), E_2 (5 pg/mL), AMH (3.1 pmol/L), and ACTH (4.2 pmol/L). Her serum prolactin level was also reduced (4.4 ng/mL), whereas her adrenal and thyroid hormone levels were normal. At ultrasonographic examination, the volumes of both her right ovary (3.5 mL) and left ovary (3.2 mL) were below the reference ranges established in normally ovulating patients. Computed tomography of the pituitary gland was normal. A normal 46,XX karyotype was confirmed. Hysterosalpingography revealed patent tubes and a normally developed uterus. The clinical presentation suggested the diagnosis of Kallmann syndrome and the patient was prescribed the combined oral contraceptive pill to induce regular menstrual bleeding and ensure adequate hormone replacement prior to undergoing further ovulation induction treatment.

Action plan

After just a month of oral contraception treatment, on the second day of the menstrual cycle the patient underwent ovarian induction treatment. As the patient did not respond adequately to hMG treatment we selected a different approach, with highly purified FSH. A total dose of 5625 IU was given over 14 days of stimulation. There was an appropriate endometrial thickening of 11 mm and three follicles with a mean diameter of >1.7 cm were obtained, after which 10 000 IU of human chorionic gonadotropin (hCG) was administered.

Intrauterine insemination was performed 36 hours after the injection of hCG. Intramuscular injections of hCG (1500 IU) were prescribed for luteal support on alternate days until serum β-hCG was assayed. A clinical pregnancy was diagnosed by ultrasound.

Discussion

The cause of the hypogonadism and anosmia that characterize Kallmann syndrome is a congenital, isolated GnRH deficiency resulting from aplasia of both GnRH-secreting cells and olfactory bulbs. The incidence of Kallmann syndrome in females is about 1:50 000, and the condition may be associated with some congenital abnormalities (e.g., cleft lip and palate, renal agenesis, cardiac anomalies, and abnormal platelet function).

Fertility therapies proposed were based on hormonal replacement of the insufficient FSH and LH secretion. The majority of pregnancies that have been reported in the literature in patients with Kallmann syndrome were achieved by the combined administration of hMG or hMG with hCG, or by the long-term administration of pulsatile GnRH through an infusion pump [1, 2].

It seems that also highly purified FSH and hCG could be used for ovarian stimulation in order to achieve a pregnancy in a woman with Kallmann syndrome [3]. The outcome of this case is not consistent with the reported need for exogenous LH during controlled ovarian stimulation (COS). However, theca cells may require very low levels of LH for appropriate folliculogenesis. Studies using recombinant FSH alone in women with no pituitary activity have shown that it is adequate for the recruitment and growth of follicles, and hCG administration may be sufficient to allow normal luteinization. In this case, the response of the endometrium to ovarian stimulation with purified FSH suggests that some level of LH activity was present. The lack of effect of hMG treatment in this patient might be explained by a mutation of the LH receptor gene.

Although ovulation induction using hMG or GnRH seems to be more reasonable, in patients with Kallmann syndrome, the use of highly purified FSH may be another option of treatment. Due to the genetic characteristics of Kallmann syndrome, which have been demonstrated to be autosomal dominant type, it is quite possible that the clinical features of this particular case could be the result of a mutation [4]. It seems that not all cases of Kallmann syndrome are classic hypogonadotropic hypogonadism and that a pragmatic approach may be useful.

References

1. Crowley WF, McArthur JW. Stimulation of the normal menstrual cycle in Kallmann's syndrome by pulsatile administration of luteinizing-releasing hormone. *J Clin Endocrinol Metab* 1980; **51**: 173–5

2. Chryssicopoulos A, Gregoriu O, Papadias C, Loghis C. Gonadotropin ovulation induction and pregnancies in women with Kallmann's syndrome. *Gynecol Endocrinol* 1998; **12**: 103–8

3. Battaglia C, Salvatori M, Regnani G, Giulini S, Primavera MR, Volpe A. Successful induction of ovulation using highly purified follicle-stimulating hormone in a woman with Kallmann's syndrome. *Fertil Steril* 2000; **2**: 284–6.

4. Dodé C, Hardelin JP. Kallmann syndrome. *Eur J Hum Genet* 2009; **17**: 139–46.

Chapter

12

A patient with severe endometriosis needing IVF

Luk Rombauts, Sameer Jatkar, Sofie Piessens, and Peter Carne

Clinical fertility history

A 27-year-old woman was referred for evaluation of 18 months' primary infertility in the setting of known severe endometriosis, first diagnosed 4 years earlier after presenting with severe dysmenorrhea and deep dyspareunia. After initial laparoscopic resection, she was treated with continuous combined contraceptive pill and a repeat laparoscopy was performed for symptom recurrence when she stopped the pill with the intention to conceive. The second laparoscopy diagnosed bilateral tubal occlusion and nodular endometriosis over the bladder, uterosacral ligaments, and sigmoid colon.

At the time of referral, the patient reported worsening dyschezia and cyclical rectal bleeding. Her main priority, however, was achieving a pregnancy through IVF.

General medical, family, and social history

The patient was a primary school teacher with no significant other past history or comorbidities apart from mild asthma requiring use of inhaled reliever medication. Her 31-year-old male partner was otherwise well with no significant past history and family history was unremarkable for both. Both partners were nonsmokers with a healthy lifestyle.

Examination findings

General examination of the patient was largely unremarkable, although pelvic examination revealed nodules consistent with endometriosis on the uterosacral ligaments. Rectal examination was unremarkable. Her BMI was 21 kg/m².

Fertility investigations

During the initial fertility workup a transvaginal ultrasound examination undertaken by an obstetric and gynecologist sonologist revealed a large endometriotic lesion on the distal sigmoid colon of at least 2.9 cm maximal diameter. The left ovary was adherent to the posterior uterus with a small 1.8-cm diameter endometrioma present on the same side.

Other fertility investigations including hormone profile and semen analysis were within normal limits. The antimüllerian hormone level of 14 pmol/L was within the normal range for her age preoperatively.

Other clinical investigations

A colonoscopy was performed but did not reveal luminal pathology.

Diagnosis

Deep infiltrating endometriosis with large-bowel involvement and tubal infertility.

Action plan

The patient elected to defer surgery and proceed to IVF in view of bilateral tubal blockage. However, with the menstrual bleed following the first unsuccessful IVF cycle the patient presented with a severe exacerbation of abdominal pain and rectal bleeding requiring hospital admission. The patient then requested a complete clearance of the pelvic endometriosis.

Outcome

The patient underwent a laparoscopic anterior resection and complete excision of deep infiltrating endometriosis (DIE). Histology of the anterior resection revealed that the endometriotic lesion infiltrated the full thickness of the colonic muscularis. The symptoms resolved completely postoperatively with satisfactory recovery of normal bowel function.

Antral follicle count prior to the next stimulated cycle was 13 and she responded well in her next IVF cycle, with transfer of two blastocysts on day 5. The patient subsequently achieved a dichorionic diamniotic twin pregnancy with healthy twins born at term.

Discussion

There is little consensus with respect to the treatment of severe endometriosis prior to IVF treatment. Endometriosis sufferers have been reported to have a significantly lowered pregnancy rate following IVF and this effect is more pronounced in those with more advanced disease. A number of treatments have been advocated for the management of severe endometriosis, including hormonal and nonhormonal medical management as well as surgical management; however, some of these are not appropriate in those patients who are trying to conceive [1].

One variant, deep infiltrating endometriosis, is reported to affect the bowel in up to 37% of women with endometriosis [2]. Intestinal endometriosis varies from superficial lesions involving the serosa only to any degree of invasion, including full thickness with erosion of the bowel mucosa. Bowel lesions predominantly affect the rectum and sigmoid colon, with a large majority of lesions found in this location in the distal 20 cm of bowel [3]. Reported complications include intestinal perforation and flares of severe pain during IVF stimulation with a worsening of frequently encountered symptoms such as cramping pelvic pain, constipation, dyschezia, and rectal bleeding.

No randomized trials have been performed to prove that surgery prior to IVF improves pregnancy rates. There is, however, high-level evidence from a systematic review that pre-IVF treatment with GnRH analogues for 3–6 months increases pregnancy rates considerably (odds ratio 4.3) in these women with severe disease [4].

Nevertheless, some patients will experience intolerable pain during ovarian stimulation despite pituitary down regulation and require surgery before they can continue with IVF. Careful preoperative planning is essential whenever bowel involvement is suspected. Transvaginal ultrasound is the most appropriate first-line imaging modality for the identification of bowel deposits, and has good sensitivity, specificity, and positive predictive value [5]. When access is available to high-quality ultrasound, MRI can be reserved for those who cannot tolerate transvaginal scanning or who are virgo intacta. Bowel preparation and the involvement of a multidisciplinary team, including a colorectal surgeon, should always be arranged to reduce the complication rate in these complex procedures.

Segmental bowel resection of endometriotic deposits can indeed relieve pain and gastrointestinal symptoms and result in an improved quality of life. Additionally, it can prevent the worsening of bowel-related symptoms during IVF stimulation while there is also some evidence from observational studies that this treatment in itself may improve fertility for both spontaneous and IVF conceptions. Among IVF patients, it has been reported that extensive laparoscopic treatment of deep infiltrating endometriosis resulted in an odds ratio of pregnancy of 2.45 compared with no endometriosis treatment [6].

However, not all bowel lesions require a segmental resection. Alternative options include "shaving" or superficial excision for those lesions that are not invading beyond the muscularis. This technique involves the superficial peeling of serosal and subserosal endometriosis or excision respectively without opening the bowel wall. Alternatively, full-thickness disk excision of the anterior rectal wall may be undertaken using a circular stapling device.

Thus, in the setting of severe endometriosis with large-bowel involvement, pre-treatment with GnRH-analog for 3–6 months may be an appropriate strategy if the pain is manageable. However, if symptoms of infiltrating disease worsen significantly during IVF treatment, surgery may become unavoidable. Such surgery is best performed laparoscopically by a multidisciplinary team following careful preoperative transvaginal ultrasound assessment.

References

1. Koch J, Rowan K, Rombauts L, Yazdani A, Chapman M, Johnson N. Endometriosis and Infertility – a consensus statement from ACCEPT (Australasian CREI Consensus Expert Panel on Trial Evidence). *Aust N Z J Obstet Gynaecol* 2012; **52**(6): 513–22.

2. Remorgida V, Ferrero S, Fulcheri E, Ragni N, Martin D. Bowel endometriosis: presentation, diagnosis, and treatment. *Obstet Gynecol Surv* 2007; **62**(7): 461–70.

3. Wills H, Reid G, Cooper M, Morgan M. Fertility and pain outcomes following laparoscopic segmental bowel resection for colorectal endometriosis: a review. *Aust N Z J Obstet Gynecol* 2008; **48**(3): 292–5.

4. Sallam H, Garcia-Velasco J, Dias S, Arici A, Abou-Setta A. Long-term pituitary down-regulation before in vitro fertilization (IVF) for women with endometriosis. *Cochrane Database Syst Rev* 2006: (1): CD004635.

5. Hudelist G, English J, Thomas A, Tinelli A, Singer C, Keckstein J. Diagnostic accuracy of transvaginal ultrasound for non-invasive diagnosis of bowel endometriosis: systematic review and meta-analysis. *Ultrasound Obstet Gynecol* 2011; **37**(3): 257–63.

6. Bianchi P, Pereira R, Zanatta A, Alegretti J, Motta E, Serafini P. Extensive excision of deep infiltrative endometriosis before in vitro fertilization significantly improves pregnancy rates. *J Minim Invasive Gynecol* 2009; **16**(2): 174–80.

Chapter

13

Recurrent miscarriage due to a balanced translocation
A case of PGS

Michael J. Paidas and S. Ornaghi

Clinical fertility history

A 35-year-old woman and her 40-year-old male partner presented for investigation with a history of three recurrent miscarriages after they had conceived naturally after only a few months of trying. The first miscarriage was around 12 weeks gestation, the second at 8 weeks, and the third at around 5–6 weeks. The first two miscarriages ended with a dilatation and curettage, however no karyotyping was performed on the products of conception. The third miscarriage was complete and did not require surgical intervention. She has a regular menstrual cycle, with no dysmenorrhea, dyspareunia, or abnormal uterine bleeding. Her only medications were folic acid.

General medical, family, and social history

The couple were of Caucasian background, and healthy; neither smoked and they infrequently used alcohol. There was no medical or family history of thrombophilia or auto-immune disease.

The male partner had no significant medical or family history.

The 35-year-old woman had a family history with one cousin having a "chromosome problem," but there was uncertainty about the family details here. Her father had died of a heart-related problem, her mother was alive and well, and the three brothers were well. On further enquiry into her brother's fertility history, all three had children but some pregnancies ended in miscarriage. She was told that one of her brothers' miscarriages was thought to be related to the wife's polycystic ovary syndrome. None of the first-degree relatives had undergone chromosome testing.

Examination findings

Examination findings were overall normal. She had a BMI of 25 kg/m²; he had a BMI of 26 kg/m².

Fertility investigations

Both partners had further investigations, including the full antenatal screening tests; full blood count, hemoglobin, hemoglobinopathy testing, iron studies, hepatitis B and C and HIV, rubella and varicella serology, VDRL test, and TSH. All were normal. The antimüllerian hormone (AMH) level was 35 pmol/L (local laboratory range 14–30 pmol/L), and her blood group was A positive.

A pelvic ultrasound showed an anteverted uterus and tubal patency testing via hystero-salpingo-contrast sonography (Hycosy) revealed patent fallopian tubes. There was no obvious uterine abnormality.

A number of tests were carried out to elucidate a possible cause for recurrent miscarriage. These included lupus anticoagulant, anti-cardiolipin antibody, Leiden V factor, protein S, protein C, antithrombin III, homocysteine, fasting glucose, fasting insulin, and chromosomes from peripheral leukocytes. Her karyotype revealed a balanced translocation involving chromosomes 11 and 22. This was reported as 46XX,t(11;22)(q23.3;q11.2), which is one of the most commonly seen translocations.

Interestingly she was also heterozygous for factor V Leiden, which can be another factor associated with increased risk of miscarriage, although conflicting results are reported in literature.

Her partner had a normal semen analysis, and sperm chromatin structure assay (SCSA) showed a DNA fragmentation index of 6.0% (normal range 1–15%). His karyotype was normal (46 XY).

Diagnosis

Balanced translocation of chromosomes 11 and 22.

Action plan

This couple described their miscarriages as "a rollercoaster of emotion." After genetic counseling, they elected to proceed with IVF/ICSI, and to undergo preimplantation genetic diagnosis (PGD) with comparative genomic hybridization (CGH) in order to screen the embryos for any unbalanced chromosomes or aneuploidy, with the aim of increasing their chance of an ongoing pregnancy and live-born baby. Of note, the patient was heterozygous for factor V Leiden mutation, but she did not have any additional thromboembolic risk factor and did not experience ovarian hyper stimulation syndrome. Therefore, prophylactic anticoagulant therapy was not administered for the IVF procedure or during the antepartum period. In recent clinical trials, prophylactic antepartum anticoagulation has not been proven beneficial in improving pregnancy outcome in women with FVL and recurrent pregnancy loss. Anticoagulation, that is low-molecular-weight heparin (Clexane [enoxaparin]) was administered in the postpartum period to reduce the maternal risk of venous thromboembolism.

The IVF cycle used was a long down regulation protocol to aid planning of oocyte retrieval and PGD. FSH 100 IU was used for ovarian stimulation. Recombinant hCG was given 36 hours before egg recovery and progesterone pessaries 200 mg twice day were used in the luteal phase for endometrial support.

Outcome

The egg retrieval was done on day 14 from the start of FSH stimulation. Eleven of the 15 eggs collected were mature, and eight fertilized.

By day 3 post egg retrieval, five of the eight embryos were of a developing stage and grade to be biopsied for CGH array PGD. Single-cell biopsies were carried out and the 24Sure+ BAC array (Bluegnome, UK) was used for the CGH analysis. The three remaining embryos not biopsied went on to fragment and ceased developing.

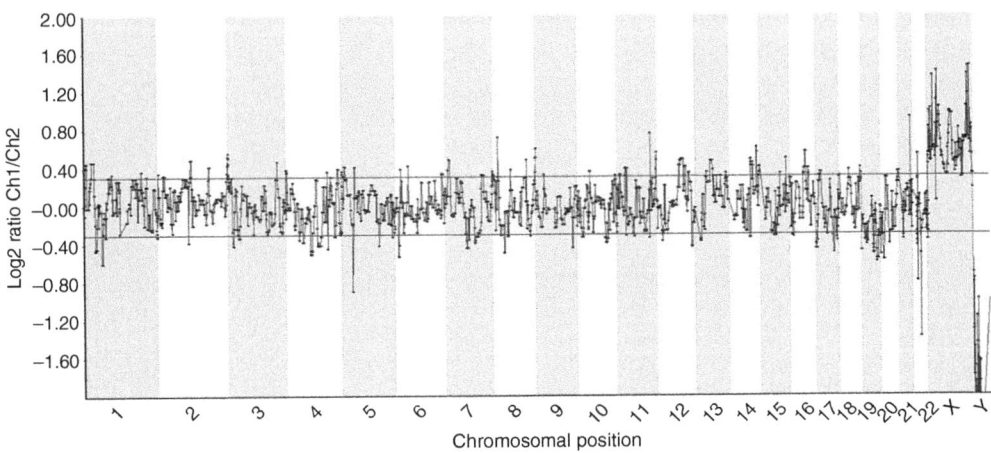

Figure 13.1 Normal female 46,XX array.

Table 13.1 PGD/CGH outcome

Embryo	Day 5	Array PGD result on biopsied cells
1	Early blastocyst	−1q
2	Hatching blastocyst	NAD
3	Early blastocyst	−3p, +11q
4	Morula	+11q, −22q
5	Hatching blastocyst	+11, −22p

On the fifth day post egg retrieval the results of the biopsied cells showed that only one of the five embryos tested was euploid. This was a "normal" blastocyst and was transferred back with ease. (See Figure 13.1 showing the normal female 46,XX array.)

The remaining four embryos were unbalanced and aneuploid (see Table 13.1 for PGD/CGH array result of the patient's embryos).

Twelve days later she had a positive pregnancy test with β-hCG levels of 377 mIU/mL and a progesterone level of 575nmol/L. One week later, levels were 9483 mIU/mL and 624 nmol/L respectively.

A 6 + 4 week ultrasound showed a single viable fetus. She was referred to an obstetrician, had a normal antenatal course, and delivered vaginally a female baby weighing 3200 g.

General remarks

This is a case of a couple presenting with a history of three recurring miscarriages. A potential contributing factor was identified in the female partner, that is a balanced translocation involving chromosomes 11 and 22, 46XX,t(11;22)(q23.3;q11.2).

It is estimated that 1 in 625 individuals carries a balanced chromosomal translocation. In couples with recurrent miscarriage, the incidence of either member of the couple being a carrier of a structural chromosome abnormality is approximately 3–4%, mainly including reciprocal translocations and robertsonian translocations [1, 2].

The decision was made to use PGD as the couple had suffered a difficult and sad time with their miscarriages and wanted the reassurance that their next pregnancy would have a reduced chance of another failure.

Carriers of balanced chromosomal translocation are at increased risk for infertility, pregnancy loss, and offspring with congenital abnormalities and mental retardation as a result of unbalanced segregation. PGD is now widely used in many fertility centers and provides an option to exclude the unbalanced and aneuploid embryos [2].

We used comparative genomic hybridization (CGH) array PGD for screening the embryos. The benefit of array PGD use in screening balanced translocations and robertsonian translocations is that the procedure involves screening the entire complement of chromosomes from a single cell. The array CGH can detect chromosome imbalances in the embryo, and also provide the benefit of aneuploidy screening of all 24 chromosomes [1].

The use of PGD for carriers of balanced translocations allows us to select out and transfer those embryos with a normal or balanced chromosome complement. It also may help to reduce the risk of recurrent miscarriage and improve live birth; however, many of the embryos produced either are unbalanced themselves or have complex aneuploidy and therefore cannot be used [2, 3, 4].

It is reported that about 20% of PGD cycles have no normal or balanced embryos to transfer. Munne et al. in their study looking at outcomes of PGD in translocation carriers found that only 18.3% of the embryos formed were genetically normal or balanced, while Fiorentino et al. showed 16% and the ESHRE PGD consortium reported that of the 24 773 embryos successfully diagnosed only 26% were suitable for transfer [2, 3, 4].

In this case one of the five embryos tested (20%) was normal. This appears consistent with the literature. Of the remaining four embryos, three had a trisomy 11 in their complement of chromosomes and two were missing chromosome 22 (see Table 13.1). If this couple had an IVF cycle without PGD, one of the chromosomally abnormal embryos, a hatching blastocyst, would have been cryopreserved for their future use, ending in a poor outcome.

In summary, the couple presented with a history of three recurring miscarriages. One of the investigations revealed a balanced translocation in the female partner involving chromosome 11 and 22. To reduce their chances of another miscarriage and further heartache they underwent an IVF and ICSI cycle with PGD and CGH analysis. Of the five embryos tested one normal embryo was transferred with a positive outcome – the birth of a healthy girl.

References

1. Wilton L. Preimplantation genetic analysis and chromosome analysis of blastomeres using comparative genomic hybridisation. *Hum Reprod Update* 2005; **11**(1): 33–41.

2. Munne S, Sandalinas M, Escudero T et al. Outcome of preimplantation genetic diagnosis of translocations. *Fertil Steril* 2000; **73**: 1209–18.

3. Harper JC, Wilton L, Traeger-Synodinos J et al. The EHRE PGD Consortium: 10 years of data collection. *Hum Reprod Update* 2012; **18**(3): 234–47.

4. Fiorentino F, Spizzichino L, Bono S et al. PGD for Reciprocal and Robertsonian translocations using array comparative genomic hybridisation. *Hum Reprod* 2011; **26**(7): 1925–35.

A patient found to have Cushing syndrome

Sunita De Sousa and Robert J. Norman

Clinical fertility history

A 35-year-old woman presented with a 2-year history of secondary infertility after having two children, conceived naturally. During this time she developed oligomenorrhea, hirsutism, and weight gain of 10 kg. She denied galactorrhea. There was no prior menstrual irregularity.

General medical, family, and social history

Past medical and family histories were unremarkable. She did not take any medications. She denied changes in diet, exercise, and stress levels and did not consume alcohol.

Examination findings

Her weight was 85 kg and BMI 27 kg/m^2 with increased abdominal girth. She had diastolic hypertension with BP 135/100. Examination revealed wide purple striae on the abdomen. There was no dorsocervical fat pad. Cardiovascular, respiratory, gastrointestinal, and gynecological examinations were unremarkable. Power, reflexes, and visual fields were normal on neurological examination.

Preliminary fertility investigations

Routine biochemistry, full blood count, and thyroid function tests were normal. Reproductive hormone levels were also unremarkable: LH 5 U/L, FSH 4 U/L, estradiol 200 pmol/L, and prolactin 400 mIU/L. DHEAS and 17-hydroxyprogesterone were normal. Early morning cortisol was within normal range at 450 nmol/L. Ultrasound demonstrated normal ovaries and uterus.

Other clinical investigations

A preliminary diagnosis of polycystic ovary syndrome was made after the above exclusion of thyroid dysfunction, hyperprolactinemia, and nonclassical congenital adrenal hyperplasia. However, she went on to have an overnight 1 mg dexamethasone suppression test, which showed elevated cortisol at 250 nmol/L at 08:00 the next day. 24-hour free urinary cortisol was also raised. ACTH was borderline high. Growth hormone and insulin-like growth factor-I were normal. Urine osmolality was normal, demonstrating intact posterior pituitary function.

A low-dose dexamethasone suppression test (0.5 mg qid for 2 days) showed no suppression, while high-dose dexamethasone (2 mg qid for 2 days) achieved suppression. MRI of the pituitary revealed a small anterior pituitary mass with no extension. Adrenal ultrasound showed hyperplasia and no nodules.

Inferior petrosal sinus sampling confirmed excess ACTH secretion from the right side of the pituitary.

Diagnosis

Hypercortisolism due to an ACTH-producing pituitary adenoma (Cushing disease).

Action plan

Transphenoidal resection of the pituitary mass was performed with a small amount of intra-operative bleeding.

Outcome

Subsequent hormonal panels showed normalization of the pituitary–adrenal axis with no evidence of hypopituitarism of the other axes. Normal menstrual cycles resumed within 4 months.

General remarks

Cushing syndrome refers to the clinical syndrome of hypercortisolism including obesity, central and supraclavicular fat deposition, hypertension, insulin resistance, myopathy, and osteoporosis. During reproductive age, affected females may present with amenorrhea, hirsutism, and infertility, all of which may be found in other diseases of infertility including the much more common polycystic ovary syndrome.

The infertility of Cushing syndrome is incompletely understood, but viable hypotheses include the hyperandrogenism of hypercortisolism suppressing gonadotropin secretion, direct antagonism of cortisol receptors on GnRH neurons, and blockade of gonadotropic effects on the gonads. Regardless of the specific mechanism, up to 80% of hypercortisolemic women have oligomenorrhea or amenorrhea. Pituitary sources of hypercortisolism appear to hamper fertility more than ACTH-independent hypercortisolism, which may be due to the stimulating effect of ACTH on the zona reticularis to make DHEA.

Hypercortisolism is established by positive results of at least two screening tests: 24-hour urinary free cortisol, late night salivary cortisol or serum cortisol coinciding with the natural nadir of cortisol secretion and the overnight low-dose dexamethasone suppression test demonstrating autonomous hormone production.

Cushing disease specifically refers to hypercortisolism due to an ACTH-producing pituitary adenoma. Such ACTH-dependence may be established by an inappropriately normal or high plasma ACTH level. Corticotropin-releasing hormone (CRH) and high-dose dexamethasone tests are subsequently performed to identify ACTH-producing adenomatous pituitary tissue which will maintain a normal stimulatory response to CRH and a normal suppressive response to high-dose dexamethasone. This is in contrast to ectopic ACTH production where the neoplastic tissue cannot be inhibited by even this higher dose of dexamethasone and pituitary responses have been blunted by the ectopic ACTH. Finally, anatomical localization of Cushing disease is usually achieved by pituitary MRI and, if inconclusive, petrosal sinus sampling to lateralize the source of ACTH.

Transphenoidal pituitary adenectomy is the mainstay of therapy for Cushing disease, with remission rates of 60–80%. This is usually sufficient for restoration of fertility, and also improves maternal and fetal outcomes in pregnancy as hypercortisolism has been associated with gestational diabetes mellitus, preeclampsia, heart failure, hypertension, myopathy, poor wound healing, premature labor, intrauterine growth retardation, and fetal loss.

Further reading

Chang AY, Auchus RJ. Endocrine disturbances affecting reproduction. In: Strauss JF, Barbieri RL (eds.). *Yen and Jaffe's Reproductive Endocrinology*, 6th edition. Philadelphia, PA: Saunders Elsevier; 2009.

Lekarev O, New MI. Adrenal disease in pregnancy. *Best Pract Res Clin Endo Metab* 2011; **25**:959–73.

Newell-Price J, Bertagna X, Grossman AB, Nieman LK. Cushing's syndrome. *Lancet* 2006; **367**:1605–17.

The Practice Committee of the American Society for Reproductive Medicine. The evaluation and treatment of androgen excess. *Fertil Steril* 2006; **86**(S4): S241–7.

Chapter

15

Postpartum pituitary problems

Tristan Hardy and Robert J. Norman

Clinical fertility history

A 32-year-old woman presented with secondary infertility of 18 months duration. She had two previous pregnancies to the same partner, both resulting in live births. The first child was delivered in a major hospital, and was successfully breast fed until the mother fell pregnant with the second, who was delivered in a peripheral center. Postnatally the patient was unable to establish breast feeding due to illness after delivery and bottle fed for 9 months. She commenced the progestin-only oral contraceptive pill and did not have a period thereafter. As she was feeling lethargic and generally unwell, she had consulted her general practitioner, who checked her thyroid status and commenced thyroxine 100 µg daily due to a low free thyroxine result.

General medical, family, and social history

The patient had no significant prior medical history, and there was no family history of infertility, recurrent pregnancy loss, autoimmune conditions, or endocrinopathies. She was in a supportive relationship and had not returned to work since the birth of her first child due to lethargy and child rearing. She had ongoing dyspareunia.

Examination findings

On examination the patient appeared overweight, with a low pulse rate, dry skin, and cold peripheries. Diminished secondary sex characteristics and signs of hypoestrogenism were noted, with reduced pubic and axillary hair and atrophic vaginal tissue. Gynecological examination revealed a small uterine size on bimanual examination. No abnormalities were detected on neurological examination, in particular no visual field defects.

Fertility investigations

An endocrine profile was performed first due to the nature of the presentation. The previous result of a low free thyroxine (FT4) was associated with low TSH and no thyroid antibodies. TSH was undetectable off thyroxine. Prolactin was undetectable (<25 U/L), FSH and LH were both low (<1 U/L), and there was biochemical evidence of hypoestrogenism (E2 < 50 pmol/L). Cranial MRI was normal, with no evidence of sellar or parasellar tumors or other lesions. She did not have a withdrawal bleed following administration of norethisterone acetate 5 mg for 5 days.

On further questioning, a history of significant postpartum hemorrhage was elicited, with more than 12 units of blood given for hypovolemic shock following her second delivery.

53

Other clinical investigations

Other clinical investigations confirmed low HGH and IGF1, very low urine/serum osmolality indicating diabetes insipidus, and low serum cortisol (50 nmol/L AM and 120 nmol/L PM). Synacthen test showed a normal response of cortisol after 60 minutes.

Diagnosis

Panhypopituitarism secondary to postpartum pituitary necrosis (Sheehan syndrome).

Action plan

The patient was started on thyroxine, hydrocortisone, and vasopressin and her symptoms improved. From a fertility perspective, she was given low-dose estrogen for 3 months prior to treatment by assisted reproductive technology in order to restore uterine size. She then underwent FSH ovulation induction with recombinant LH added when follicle size reached 10 mm, and hCG administered when follicle size reached 17 mm.

No additional luteal phase medications were added.

Outcome

FSH ovulation induction was successful, with the patient conceiving within two cycles. She went on to have a normal vaginal delivery at term.

General remarks

Sheehan syndrome refers to postpartum hypopituitarism usually resulting from massive obstetric hemorrhage. The anterior pituitary is thought to be particularly prone to infarction and necrosis in pregnancy due to hypertrophy of pituitary lactotrophs, which may cause compression of blood vessels and may be particularly sensitive to ischemia. Although a rare cause of hypopituitarism compared with pituitary neoplasms, it remains an important differential in the reproductive-age population and has a range of clinical presentations from immediate, life-threatening deficiencies of adrenocorticotropic, thyroid-stimulating, and antidiuretic hormones to subclinical, chronic deficiencies of growth hormone or gonadotropins. Hormone replacement therapy is required both in the short term and to avoid the long-term chronic morbidities associated with hypopituitarism.

In women presenting to fertility clinics, symptoms related to gonadotropin deficiency may include oligoamenorrhea, loss of libido, dyspareunia, and infertility. Although spontaneous pregnancies in patients with Sheehan syndrome have been reported, the majority will require some form of assisted reproductive technology to achieve a pregnancy. Induction of ovulation with recombinant FSH can be expected to restore near normal fecundity. Addition of LH is essential once the follicle starts to grow as it provides the androgens required for aromatization to estrogens. Use of the oral contraceptive pill, estradiol valerate, or transdermal estradiol patches is recommended prior to fertility treatment to restore uterine volume.

Pregnancies resulting from fertility treatment for hypopituitarism remain at high risk of miscarriage, stillbirth, and intrauterine growth restriction, especially with multiple gestations, probably due to poor placental function. This reinforces the importance of follicle tracking and strict cancellation criteria in these patients to avoid multiple pregnancy, and adequate uterine preparation prior to pregnancy with estrogen replacement therapy. Luteal phase support with progesterone suppositories has sometimes been recommended to reduce the risk of early pregnancy loss. Awareness of these strategies is important not only in the case of patients with Sheehan syndrome, and can be applied to any patient requiring ovulation induction for hypopituitarism.

Further reading

Kovacs K. Sheehan syndrome. *Lancet* 2003; **361**: 520–2.

Overton CE, Davis CJ, West, C, Davies MC, Conway GS. High risk pregnancies in hypopituitary women. *Human Reproduction* 2002; **17**(6): 1464–7.

Schneider HJ, Aimaretti G, Kreitschmann-Andermahr I, Stalla G, Ghigo E. Hypopituitarism. *Lancet* 2007; **369**(9571): 146–70.

Large bilateral endometriomas

Juan A. Garcia-Velasco and Israel Ortega

Clinical fertility history

A 34-year-old woman had been trying to conceive for two years. She had not been pregnant before and had not undergone any previous fertility treatment. Her partner had normal sperm parameters but her hysterosalpingogram revealed bilateral tubal blockage. At vaginal ultrasonography, bilateral endometriomas of 5 and 6 cm were observed. She reported mild dysmenorrhea but no other symptoms of endometriosis. She was advised to undergo surgery for her bilateral, asymptomatic endometriomas prior to commencing fertility treatment.

General medical, family, and social history

Her father had had colon cancer successfully operated a few years previously. Her mother had had the thyroid removed and was being treated for hypertension. Her sister had one daughter and also had an endometrioma removed prior to her spontaneous pregnancy. The patient not drink or smoke, and was not taking any medication. Her last pap smear less than a year previously showed no significant findings.

Examination findings

Physical examination was unremarkable. Her height and weight were 1.68 m and 59 kg, respectively, resulting in a body mass index (BMI) in the normal range (20.9 kg/m^2). No masses were palpated on either abdominal or bimanual examination.

Fertility investigations

The results of her laboratory endocrine evaluation carried out on the third day of her menstruation were: PRL, 25 ng/mL; TSH, 2.3 mIU/L; FSH, 12 mIU/mL; estradiol, 56 pg/mL; AMH, 8.36 pmol/L.

Hysterosalpingography for evaluation of tubal patency showed bilateral tubal blockage. Mock embryo transfer procedures were uncomplicated.

A transvaginal ultrasound scan showed a normal-shaped uterus, 5.9 × 2.0 × 3.2 cm in size, anteflexed, homogenic normal echostructure, and a regular endometrium of 8.8 mm. The right ovary contained a well-circumscribed, thick-walled cyst of 5 cm characterized by homogeneous low-level internal echoes compatible with endometrioma. The left ovary showed a cyst of similar characteristics up to 6 cm. The antral follicle count (of follicles measuring 2–9 mm) was 2 in the left ovary and 1 in the right ovary. No free fluid was observed in the pouch of Douglas. Three-dimensional power Doppler imaging demonstrated normal ovarian blood flow.

Magnetic resonance imaging showed the uterosacral ligaments, adnexae, rectovaginal septum, urinary bladder, and the wall of the rectosigmoid colon to be otherwise free of endometriotic nodules or solid masses and ruled out the presence of deep invasive endometriosis.

Semen analysis showed normal parameters, such as a sperm count of 21 million/mL, progressive motility of 40%, and morphology of 6%.

Other clinical investigations

Laboratory workup reported the following levels: hemoglobin 13.6 g/dL, hematocrit 45%, neutrophils 44.4%, eosinophils 7.3%. Blood chemistry showed total cholesterol 212 mg/dL, triglycerides 145 mg/dL, and very low density-cholesterol 82 mg/dL. No changes in coagulation parameters were observed. Negative serologic tests for HIV, HCV, and HBV were reported and the blood group of both partners was A+.

Diagnosis

Primary infertility due to tubal disease and severe endometriosis with low ovarian reserve.

Action plan

Controlled ovarian hyperstimulation (COH) was performed for *in vitro* fertilization (IVF). As a low response was predicted, egg vitrification was suggested to accumulate eggs until an appropriate number of oocytes was achieved in order to offer a good chance of embryo transfer. After completion of a second COH, a mixed IVF-ICSI cycle was performed, thawing the cryopreserved oocytes and fertilizing both fresh and thawed eggs. No surgical treatment of the endometriomas was performed prior to IVF treatment.

Outcome

The patient received an oral contraceptive pill (OCP) with 0.030 mg of ethinyl estradiol and 0.150 mg of levonorgestrel (Microgynon) for 14 days during the cycle before ovarian stimulation. After completion of OCP treatment, a vaginal ultrasound scan was performed to exclude the presence of any cyst or residual corpus luteum, and ovarian stimulation was started on day 5 post pill with 225 IU/day subcutaneously (SC) of rFSH (GonalF) and 75 IU/day SC of HP hMG (Menopur). On stimulation day 6, 0.25 mg of the GnRH antagonist cetrorelix (Cetrotide) was started daily and continued until the end of stimulation. Recombinant hCG alpha, 250 µg SC (Ovitrelle) was administered when at least two follicles reached 18 mm in diameter, and oocyte retrieval was scheduled 36 hours later. Two MII oocytes were retrieved on day 11 and vitrified. At the onset of menses, OCP was started again and the patient underwent a similar stimulation protocol in the subsequent cycle, retrieving two MII oocytes at ovum pick-up day. After applying standard ICSI procedure to the fresh and thawed oocytes, two out of four oocytes fertilized (one fresh and one thawed) and two 8-cell embryos were transferred on day 3 of the cleavage state. The luteal phase was supplemented with 400 mg/day of vaginal micronized progesterone (Progeffik). A pregnancy test (serum β-hCG determination) was positive 12 days later (120 IU), and a single sac with positive heartbeat was observed on week 6. Pregnancy was ongoing at 22 weeks. Figure 16.1 and 16.2 show the two endometriomas persisting at ultrasound in early pregnancy.

General remarks

Endometriosis is a common gynecological condition that affects approximately 10–15% of the female population during their reproductive years and 10–25% of patients requiring assisted reproduction technology (ART). Endometriotic ovarian cysts may be present in up to 20–40% of women with endometriosis scheduled for IVF, whereas bilateral endometriomas may represent 19–28% of cases [1, 2]. The best medical approach to treat endometriotic ovarian cysts is controversial, and whether there is any benefit or not of removing endometriomas prior to IVF remains a matter of debate.

Previously, it has been shown that laparoscopic surgical removal of ovarian endometriotic cysts prior to IVF not only damages ovarian reserve and impairs the responsiveness to hyperstimulation, but also does not offer any additional benefit in terms of fertility outcomes [3, 4]. Moreover, this damage becomes of particular clinical relevance in women with bilateral disease, since the excision of ovarian endometriomas may result in a severe impairment of the ovarian reserve and even ovarian failure [5, 6]. In addition, it should be taken into account that surgery exposes women to dangerous risks inevitably related to a demanding surgery.

In the present case report, the presence of low ovarian reserve, the lack of pain symptoms, and the absence of sonographic features of malignancy supported an expectant management of bilateral endometriomas before undergoing IVF. We have previously demonstrated that the number of developing follicles and the number of oocytes retrieved are significantly lower in women with bilateral endometriomas compared with control, leading to a decreased response to ovarian hyperstimulation [7]. However, this did not translate into significant differences in terms of number of embryos obtained and chances of pregnancy. Indeed, the rate of oocytes retrieved per total number of developing follicle, and the fertilization and implantation rates were comparable between women with bilateral endometriomas and the control group. Therefore, in spite of a poorer responsiveness to hyperstimulation in

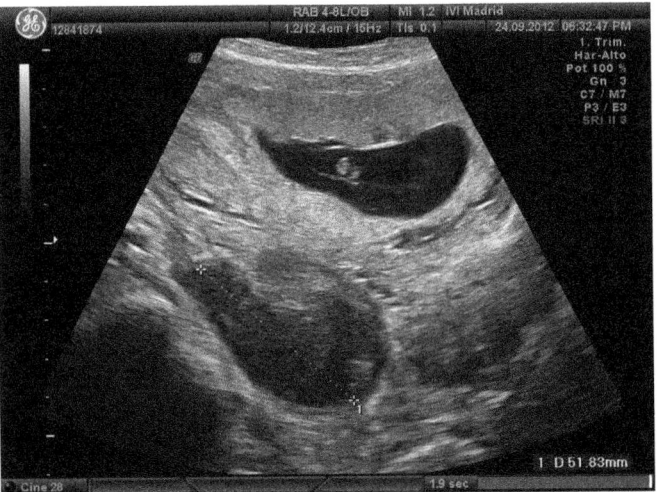

Figure 16.1 Figures 16.1 and 16.2 show the two endometriomas persisting at ultrasound in early pregnancy.

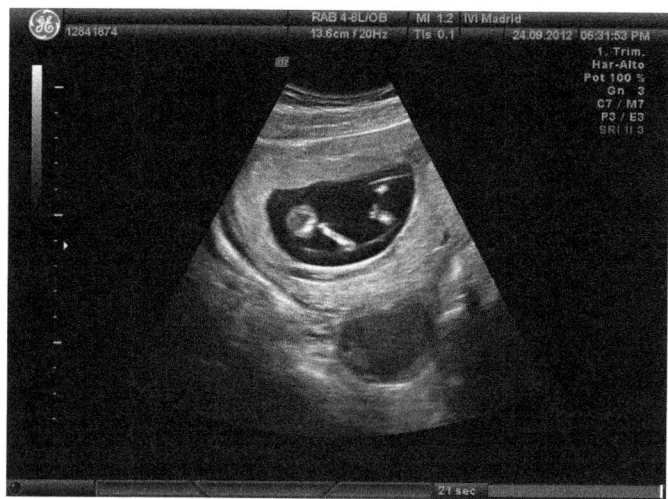

Figure 16.2

women with bilateral endometriomas, the quality of the oocytes retrieved and the chances of pregnancy are not affected.

In conclusion, the laparoscopic surgical removal of bilateral endometriomas prior to IVF should be limited to those cases with normal ovarian reserve, presence of pain symptoms, rapid growth or sonographic features of malignancy. Conversely, in the absence of the above-mentioned clinical variables, patients with bilateral endometriomas should be encouraged to proceed directly to IVF to reduce time to pregnancy, to avoid potential surgical complications and to limit costs.

References

1. Vercellini P, Chapron C, De Giorgi O, Consonni D, Frontino G, Crosignani PG. Coagulation or excision of ovarian endometriomas? *Am J Obstet Gynecol* 2003; **188**: 606–10.

2. Jenkins S, Olive DL, Haney AF. Endometriosis: pathogenetic implications of the anatomic distribution. *Obstet Gynecol* 1986; **67**: 335–8.

3. Garcia-Velasco JA, Somigliana E. Management of endometriomas in women requiring IVF: to touch or not to touch. *Hum Reprod* 2009; **24**: 496–501.

4. Somigliana E, Berlanda N, Benaglia L, Vigano P, Vercellini P, Fedele L. Surgical excision of endometriomas and ovarian reserve: a systematic review on serum antimullerian hormone level modifications. *Fertil Steril* 2012; **98**(6): 1531–8

5. Di Prospero F, Micucci G. Is operative laparoscopy safe in ovarian endometriosis? *Reprod Biomed Online* 2009;**18**: 167.

6. Somigliana E, Arnoldi M, Benaglia L, Iemmello R, Nicolosi AE, Ragni G. IVF-ICSI outcome in women operated on for bilateral endometriomas. *Hum Reprod* 2008;**23**: 1526–30.

7. Benaglia L, Bermejo A, Somigliana E, Faulisi S, Ragni G, Fedele L, García-Velasco JA. IVF outcome in women with unoperated bilateral endometriomas. *Fertil Steril* 2013; **99**: 1714–19.

A patient with a thin endometrium

Dimitra Kyrou

Clinical fertility history

A 37-year-old woman, gravida 2, para 0, and her partner presented with secondary infertility due to a tubal factor.

General medical history

The patient had undergone two dilatation and curettage procedures in order to induce first-trimester abortion 5 years previously.

The couple had undergone one previous IVF attempt at our clinic, using a GnRH antagonist protocol and 200 IU of rec FSH daily for stimulation. On day 8 of stimulation, 12 follicles of ≥14 mm were visualized; however, the endometrium was hyperechogenic and no more than 4 mm in thickness despite an estradiol concentration of 1600 pmol/L. Two days later, follicular development had met the criteria to trigger final oocyte maturation and 10 000 IU of hCG was administered. Follicular aspiration took place 36 hours later. Eight oocytes were retrieved; five were fertilized and three embryos were transferred on day 3. At that time the endometrium remained at 4 mm. For luteal support, 600 mg of vaginal micronized progesterone and 2 mg of micronized estradiol were given 3 times daily, starting on the day of follicular aspiration until pregnancy test. Unfortunately, the test was negative.

A hysteroscopy was performed and Ashermann syndrome was diagnosed. Hysteroscopic resection of intrauterine adhesions was performed.

For her second trial, 2 months later, the patient was down regulated with GnRH agonist starting in the mid luteal phase of her previous menstrual cycle, and stimulated with 300 IU hMG daily. In an attempt to increase exposure of the endometrium to estrogen and hence induce greater proliferation, 2 mg of estradiol valerate was also administered 3 times daily, starting on the first day of stimulation. An ultrasound examination on day 10 of stimulation revealed 14 follicles and an endometrium of 4 mm in thickness. hCG 10 000 IU to trigger final oocyte maturation was administered in the evening of the following day and follicular aspiration took place 36 hours later. Ten oocytes were retrieved; seven were fertilized, three embryos were transferred on day 3, and four were cryopreserved. At that time the endometrium remained at 4 mm (Figure 17.1). The patient received the same luteal support as in the previous attempt. No pregnancy was achieved.

Two months later, the patient decided to undergo a frozen-thaw embryo transfer. The preparation of the endometrium was started and continued for 14 days with 100 mg of transdermal E_2 patches every 3 days and 2 mg vaginal estradiol valerate 4 times per day. The patient also received sildenafil suppositories, at a dosage of 25 mg four times per day beginning with the initiation of estradiol administration. On day 14 of the artificial cycle,

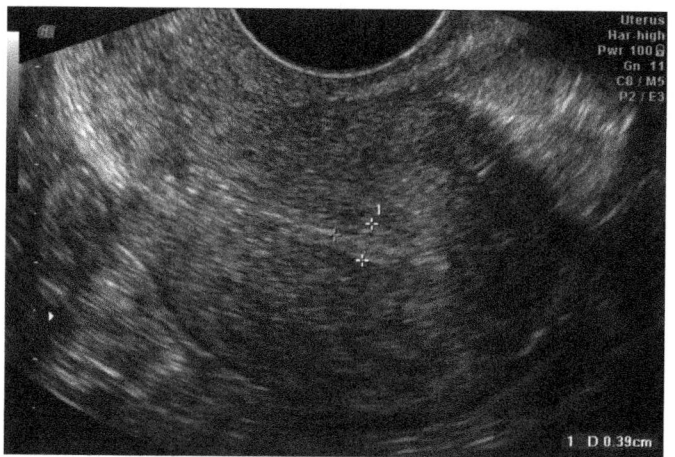

Figure 17.1 Transvaginal ultrasound scan performed on the day of oocyte pick up showed a thin endometrium of just 3.9 mm.

endometrial thickness was 4.8 mm. Embryo transfer was performed despite the low endometrial thickness after thawing of two embryos on day 3 of treatment with micronized vaginal progesterone. Unfortunately, again no pregnancy was achieved.

For her last attempt of frozen embryo transfer we proposed that empirical treatment with granulocyte colony-stimulating factor (G-CSF) be attempted. The endometrium was artificial prepared as described previously and on day 12 of preparation 300 µg/L of G-CSF was administrated into the endometrial cavity. Endometrial thickness reached 4.7 mm within 48 hours from G-CSF infusion. Embryo transfer was performed, without conception.

The patient decided to proceed to a gestational surrogacy after repeated failures to improve the endometrium.

Discussion

Embryo implantation represents the final key step which determines the success of IVF. One factor that may affect embryo implantation is uterine receptivity expressed as endometrial thickness. Although pregnancies have been reported with thin endometria, studies suggest an increased chance of implantation when the endometrial thickness is greater than 7 mm and further improvement when it is >9 mm [1, 2]. In approximately 1% of all IVF cycles, a thin endometrium is thought to underly implantation failure, and is often unresponsive to treatment [3]. Interventions are aimed at increasing thickness either raising estrogen levels, increasing endometrial blood flow, or reducing putative oxygen free radicals. While the rationale for these treatments is not supported by experimental data, low-dose aspirin [4], extended estrogen administration [5], vaginal sildenafil citrate [6], pentoxifylline [7], and G-CSF [8] are employed for the management of thin endometrium with the aim of increasing the pregnancy and implantation rates in assisted reproductive technology cycles.

These various recent modalities proposed for the treatment of thin endometrium have not been shown to be effective from an evidence-based medicine point of view. Until a better understanding of the pathophysiology and significance of the thin endomterium is reached, developing an effective treatment will remain a challenge. Moreover, well-designed prospective randomized controlled trials of any novel putative treatments will be required if better management options for the thin endometrium in ART are to be defined.

References

1. Isaacs JD, Wells CS, Williams DB, Odem RR, Gast MJ, Strickler RC. Endometrial thickness is a valid monitoring parameter in cycles of ovulation induction with metropins alone. *Fertil Steril* 1996; **65**: 262–6.

2. Weissman A, Gotlieb L, Casper RF. The detrimental effect of increased endometrial thickness on implantation and pregnancy rates and outcome in in vitro fertilization program. *Fertil Steril* 1999; **71**: 147–9.

3. Al-Ghamdi A, Coskun S, Al-Hassan S, Al-Rejjal R, Awartani K. The correlation between endometrial thickness and outcome of in vitro fertilization and embryo transfer (IVF-ET) outcome. *Reprod Biol Endocinol* 2008; **6**: 37.

4. Weckstein LN, Jacobson A, Galen D, Hampton K, Hammel J. Low-dose aspirin for oocyte donation recipients with a thin endometrium: prospective randomized study. *Fertil Steril* 1997; **68**: 927–30.

5. Chen MJ, Yang JH, Peng FH, Chen Su, Ho HN, Yang YS. Extended estrogen administration for women with thin endometrium in frozen-thawed in-vitro fertilization. *J Assist Reprod Genet* 2006; **23**: 337–42.

6. Sher G, Fisch JD. Effect of vaginal sildenafil on the outcome of in vitro fertilization (IVF) after multiple failures attributed to poor endometrial development. *Fertil Steril* 2002; **78**: 1073–6.

7. Lédée-Bataille N, Olivennes F, Lefaix JL, Chaouat G, Frydman R, Delanian S. Combined treatment by pentoxifylline and tocopherol for recipient women with a thin endometrium enrolled in an oocyte donation programme. *Hum Reprod* 2002; **17**: 1249–53.

8. Gleicher N, Vidali A. Barad DH.Successful treatment of unresponsive thin endometrium.*Fertil Steril* 2011; **6**: 2123.

A poor responder

Katrina Rowan

Clinical fertility history

Ms. P., aged 38, was referred from her general gynecologist after 12 months of trying to conceive. Just prior to trying to conceive, she had an abdominal myomectomy via Pfannenstiel incision for an enlarged multi-fibroid uterus that was causing menorrhagia and pressure symptoms. The pelvis was inspected at the time and there was no evidence of endometriosis. Her menstrual cycles had been regular since ceasing oral contraception, the interval ranging between 26 and 27 days. She did not suffer from any symptoms of hyperandrogenism or estrogen deficiency. Intercourse was regular in the ovulatory window and there was no sexual dysfunction for either partner.

General medical, family, and social history

There was no other relevant medical or family history for either partner. Both partners had professional careers with a moderate to high level of work stress but there were no other lifestyle concerns.

Examination findings

Ms. P. was 165 cm in height and weighed 58 kg (BMI 21.3 kg/m^2). There was no hirsutism or acne. Pelvic examination was not performed as she had had a laparotomy 12 months previously and her Pap smear was up to date and normal. Her partner was also of normal weight and had normal, approximately 20 mL testes bilaterally with bilateral vas deferens and there was no evidence of a clinically palpable varicocele.

Fertility investigations

Pelvic ultrasound with sonohysterogram and hysterosalpingo-contrast sonography (Hycosy) showed there were several fibroids remaining, all less than 3 cm in diameter and all in an intramural or subserosal position without cavity distortion. Tubal patency was demonstrated bilaterally. Semen analysis by WHO 2002 criteria showed a normal seminal fluid volume, normal sperm count and motility, and normal morphology.

Ms. P.'s endocrine profile on day 2 of her cycle was as follows (normal range in parentheses): FSH 6.0 U/L (2.0–13.0), LH 4.5 U/L (2.5–13.0), estradiol 102 pmol/L (<400), TSH 1.13 mU/L, prolactin 255 mIU/L (85–500), antimüllerian hormone 1.0 pmol/L (15–30). A midluteal progesterone level confirmed ovulation at 36 nmol/L (>15). A karyotype was performed in both partners and this was normal (46,XX and 46,XY).

Other clinical investigations

Routine prenatal and infectious serology was performed and this was unremarkable.

Diagnosis

A 38-year-old with primary unexplained subfertility, with a likely low ovarian reserve.

Action plan

Treatment options of expectant management, stimulated intrauterine insemination, or IVF were discussed. Given Ms. P.'s age of 38 and low ovarian reserve markers, it was decided to embark on IVF.

For the first cycle of IVF, Ms. P. underwent an antagonist cycle with 225 units of recombinant FSH, and the cycle was monitored with serial transvaginal ultrasonography and serum estradiol levels. The serum estradiol reached a peak of 2550 pmol/L on day 11 and there were three follicles over 17 mm in diameter on the day of trigger with 250 IU of rec-hCG. At oocyte retrieval, only two oocytes were collected, one of which showed signs of fertilization following IVF. The embryo was transferred on day 2 at a 4-cell stage and luteal support was given (hCG 1500 IU on days 2 and 6 after ovum pick-up). Serum hCG testing was negative on the menstrual due date.

In the next cycle Ms. P. underwent a long down regulation cycle with intranasal nafarelin acetate and 300 units of recombinant FSH. In this cycle, serum estradiol reached a peak of 6231 pmol/L and on day 10 of stimulation there were four follicles over 17 mm in diameter. A trigger of 10 000 units of U-hCG (Pregnyl) was administered. Two mature and two germinal vesicle oocytes were retrieved at ovum pick-up. One of the mature oocytes fertilized but it did not progress to cleavage stage and was not transferred into the uterus.

For her third IVF cycle, Ms. P. underwent another antagonist cycle with 300 units of recombinant FSH. Recombinant growth hormone was used in a dosage of 8 IU from day 7 of stimulation to the day after trigger. On day 11 of the cycle the peak estradiol reached 8009 pmol/L and on ultrasound there were five follicles over 17 mm in diameter, and a trigger of 250 IU of rec-hCG (Ovidrel) was administered. Six oocytes were retrieved at oocyte collection and fertilized with IVF. Five of these displayed two pronuclei at fertilization check. On day 3, all five were at a cleavage stage and the embryos were grown to blastocyst stage. On day 5, a single hatching blastocyst was transferred into the uterus. There were no other embryos suitable for cryopreservation. Luteal support was given with vaginal progesterone gel. A serum hCG 9 days post embryo transfer was positive, at a level of 118.5 IU/L.

Outcome

Ms. P. proceeded to have a normal pregnancy. A healthy female infant was delivered at term by elective cesarean section, which was planned due to her previous myomectomy.

General remarks

There has been much debate regarding the definition of a poor responder to IVF treatment. In 2011, an ESHRE consensus committee published the Bologna criteria for poor ovarian response, which they defined as either a poor ovarian response to two cycles of IVF with maximum stimulation; or two out of three of the following criteria: maternal age over 40 or risk factor for premature ovarian failure; a previous poor ovarian response (<3 oocytes) to a conventional IVF stimulation protocol; or an abnormal ovarian reserve test [1]. Ms. P. fits this definition on the latter two criteria.

Many strategies have been attempted to improve the outcomes of IVF in poor responders. A Cochrane review addressing type of pituitary down regulation protocol, use of gonadotropins or clomiphene, or adjuvant therapies such as the oral contraceptive pill, steroids, progestins, or L-arginine, failed to find any evidence to support any particular intervention for poor responders [2]. Another systematic review of 22 trials assessed the impact of several interventions for poor responders including various stimulation protocols, addition of growth hormone, transdermal testosterone, and letrozole, natural cycle IVF, recombinant vs. urinary LH, type of fertilization method, and timing of embryo transfer. This review found that there was some evidence supporting improved outcomes with the addition of growth hormone, and transfer of an embryo on day 2 compared with day 3 in poor responders [3].

A separate Cochrane review addressing the use of growth hormone in IVF demonstrated no benefit in unselected IVF cases, but a statistically significant increase in pregnancy rates in women considered poor responders (OR 3.28, 95% CI 1.74 to 6.20) [4]. There was a trend toward improved live birth rates in poor responders but this did not reach statistical significance, possibly due to inadequate power as numbers were very small and confidence intervals wide (n = 38, OR 5.81, 95% CI 0.67 to 50.39). A further meta-analysis, including an additional randomized trial with live birth data, confirmed an increase in pregnancy rate and also found a statistically significant increase in live birth rate with the use of growth hormone in poor responders (OR 3.15, 95% CI 1.26 to 7.85). The absolute increase in live birth rate was 17%, NNT = 6. Both the Cochrane review and Kolibianakis's meta-analysis commented that there was significant clinical heterogeneity in included studies; in particular, the ideal dosage regime is yet to be established.

The addition of adjuvant androgens has also been proposed as an intervention for improving the outcomes in poor responders. Dehydroepiandrosterone (DHEA), in particular, is used as an adjunct for poor responders by up to a quarter of IVF specialists worldwide [5]. Despite its widespread use, a recent systematic review and meta-analysis concluded there was insufficient evidence for use of DHEA in poor responders [6]. This same review was unable to demonstrate evidence of benefit for aromatase inhibitors, addition of rLH or hCG. Based on the pooled results of two trials, pretreatment with transdermal testosterone was associated with an increase in pregnancy and live birth rates in poor responders [6].

The decision to treat Ms. P. with growth hormone after two cycles with a poor response was made on the basis of the limited evidence of benefit, with full informed consent regarding the uncertainties and potential hazards of this treatment. The cost of growth hormone has been another factor limiting its use, but fortunately this was within affordability limits for Ms. P. DHEA and was considered for use in this case, but it was decided against due to lack of evidence of benefit. The meta-analysis demonstrating an apparent benefit for the use of transdermal testosterone had not yet been published at the time of Ms. P.'s treatment. It remains possible that the improvement in oocyte numbers, embryo development, and pregnancy outcome for Ms. P. was due to chance alone. In an analysis of inter-cycle variability, up to a third of women categorized as low or high responders had a normal response in a subsequent cycle with no change in stimulation regime [7]. This highlights the need for high-quality randomized trials to further our knowledge on how best to improve the outcomes for women who are poor responders to IVF.

References

1. Ferraretti AP, La Marca A, Fauser BCJM, Tarlatzis B, Nargund G, Gianaroli L et al. ESHRE consensus on the definition of "poor response" to ovarian stimulation for in vitro fertilization: the Bologna criteria. *Hum Reprod* 2011; **26**(7): 1616–24.

2. Pandian Z, McTavish AR, Aucott L, Hamilton MP, Bhattacharya S. Interventions for "poor responders" to controlled ovarian hyper stimulation (COH) in in-vitro fertilisation (IVF). *Cochrane Database Syst Rev* 2010; (1): CD004379.

3. Kyrou D, Kolibianakis EM, Venetis CA, Papanikolaou EG, Bontis J, Tarlatzis BC. How to improve the probability of pregnancy in poor responders undergoing in vitro fertilization: a systematic review and meta-analysis. *Fertil Steril* 2009; **91**(3): 749–66.

4. Duffy JM, Ahmad G, Mohiyiddeen L, Nardo LG, Watson A. Growth hormone for in vitro fertilization. *Cochrane Database Syst Rev* 2010; (1): CD000099.

5. Sunkara SK, Coomarasamy A, Arlt W, Bhattacharya S. Should androgen supplementation be used for poor ovarian response in IVF? *Hum Reprod* 2012; **27**(3): 637–40.

6. Bosdou JK, Venetis CA, Kolibianakis EM, Toulis KA, Goulis DG, Zepiridis L et al. The use of androgens or androgen-modulating agents in poor responders undergoing in vitro fertilization: a systematic review and meta-analysis. *Hum Reprod Update* 2012; **18**(2): 127–45.

7. Griesinger G, Rombauts L, Van Kuijk J, Mannaerts B. Intercycle variability of the ovarian response in patients undergoing repeated stimulation with corifollitropin alfa in a GnRH antagonist protocol. *Hum Reprod* **27** (suppl 2): ii302–37.

Further reading

Bosdou JK, Venetis CA, Kolibianakis EM, Toulis KA, Goulis DG, Zepiridis L et al. The use of androgens or androgen-modulating agents in poor responders undergoing in vitro fertilization: a systematic review and meta-analysis. *Hum Reprod Update* 2012; **18**(2): 127–45.

Duffy JM, Ahmad G, Mohiyiddeen L, Nardo LG, Watson A. Growth hormone for in vitro fertilization. *Cochrane Database Syst Rev* 2010; (1): CD000099.

Ferraretti AP, La Marca A, Fauser BCJM, Tarlatzis B, Nargund G, Gianaroli L et al. ESHRE consensus on the definition of "poor response" to ovarian stimulation for in vitro fertilization: the Bologna criteria. *Hum Reprod* 2011 ;**26**(7): 1616–24.

Kolibianakis E, Venetis C, Diedrich K, Tarlatzis B, Griesinger G. Addition of growth hormone to gonadotrophins in ovarian stimulation of poor responders treated by in-vitro fertilization: a systematic review and meta-analysis. *Hum Reprod Update* 2009; **15**(6): 613–22.

Pandian Z, McTavish AR, Aucott L, Hamilton MP, Bhattacharya S. Interventions for "poor responders" to controlled ovarian hyper stimulation (COH) in in-vitro fertilisation (IVF). *Cochrane Database Syst Rev* 2010; (1): CD004379.

Sallam HN, Garcia-Velasco JA, Dias S, Arici A. Long-term pituitary down-regulation before in vitro fertilization (IVF) for women with endometriosis. *Cochrane Database Syst Rev.* 2006; (1): CD004635.

Recurrent implantation failure

P. Donoso and P. Sanhueza

Clinical fertility history

A 36-year-old woman patient married to a 32-year-old man presented with a history of 3-year primary infertility. The couple had previously undergone four intrauterine insemination cycles with ovarian stimulation, developing two to three follicles, but had failed to conceive. Two fresh IVF cycles were subsequently conducted over a period of 12 months and showed a normal response to ovarian hyperstimulation (12–15 cumulus–oocyte complexes) with antagonist protocol and recombinant FSH. Additionally two frozen–thawed embryo replacements were performed after each fresh IVF cycle. IVF was performed in all cycles with a normal fertilization rate. Two high-grade embryos were transferred on each fresh trial without pregnancy and a total of five high-grade embryos were replaced on the frozen–thawed cycles without success. All embryos were replaced on day 3.

General medical, family, and social history

The patient and her partner had no background of medical disease or allergies. Her menstrual cycles were regular (28–30 days) without dysmenorrhea. There was no history of premature ovarian failure or breast and gynecological malignant disease. The patient started antidepressive medication after the second IVF failure (Sertraline 50 mg/day). The male partner had no history of cryptorchidism or genital infections.

Examination findings

Patient: Normal general physical examination. BMI 21 kg/m². Vulval and vaginal examination showed no pathological findings. Cervix and uterus were also normal. Adnexal examination showed no enlargement or pain.

Partner: Normal general physical examination. BMI 25 kg/m². Physical examination showed normal testicular size and both vasa deferentia were present.

Fertility investigations

Two-dimensional ultrasound and hysterosalpingography showed normal findings. The female endocrine profile was within normal limits (thyroid, prolactin, and mid-luteal phase progesterone). Ovarian reserve tests were normal (basal FSH 7.8 IU/L; antral follicle count 12; AMH 1.8 ng/mL). Semen analysis showed normal parameters: 35 million/mL; 52.5 million total count; 42% progressive motile sperm; 6% normal morphology (WHO criteria). Total motile sperm counts were above 10 million in all intrauterine insemination cycles.

Other clinical investigations

The patient had diagnostic laparoscopy and hysteroscopy after the three failed intrauterine inseminations. These showed normality.

Diagnosis

Unexplained primary infertility with recurrent implantation failure.

Action plan

A three-dimensional ultrasound assessment of the uterine cavity was performed, and the couple's karyotypes were investigated [1]. In addition, her ovarian reserve was reassessed and further IVF was planned to include blastocyst (rather than day 3) transfer [2, 3].

Outcome

Three-dimensional ultrasound and karyotype studies were normal. Ovarian reserve tests also showed normal results. The couple underwent a third IVF trial with blastocyst transfer. Two top-quality blastocysts were replaced, resulting in a single pregnancy delivering a healthy girl.

General remarks

Recurrent implantation failure may be identified after three failed IVF cycles or after the transfer of 10 high-grade embryos [4]. Multiple factors may contribute to embryo implantation failure, such as parental chromosomal translocations, abnormal uterine anatomy (septa, submucous myoma, or intrauterine adhesions), hydrosalpinx, or inadequate culture conditions or embryo transfer technique [5].

Some studies have suggested that local injury of the endometrium by means of a catheter or hysteroscopy can induce an inflammatory response that may facilitate the preparation for implantation [6, 7]. However, large studies are required before this can be warranted in routine clinical practice.

The artificial rupture of the zona pellucida, known as assisted hatching, has been proposed to improve implantation and clinical pregnancies [8]. A recent meta-analysis of five studies reported a significant improvement in clinical pregnancy when performed in fresh embryos transferred to women with recurrent implantation failure. However, due to the small sample size of the included studies, this meta-analysis was not able to draw any conclusions regarding live birth or miscarriage rates [9]. The only randomized controlled study evaluating preimplantation genetic aneuploidy screening as a strategy to improve recurrent implantation failure patients outcome showed no significant difference on clinical pregnancy rates [10].

A few studies have reported that congenital and acquired prothrombotic conditions are more prevalent in women with recurrent implantation failure [11]. Therefore, a possible beneficial effect of the administration of low-molecular-weight heparin (LMWH) and mini-dosage of aspirin on patients with thrombophilia and recurrent implantation failure has been discussed [5]. Nevertheless, no randomized studies have been conducted to test this hypothesis.

Finally, another possible strategy is to extend embryo culture to the blastocyst stage, aiming to improve embryo selection and uterine receptivity. Two randomized studies observed a higher implantation, pregnancy rate [2] and live birth rate per cycle [3] when a blastocyst had been replaced.

In conclusion, there is no single strategy to improve live birth rates in patients with recurrent implantation failure. Consequently, a case-by-case analysis is recommended assessing all possible etiologies and discussing the different available approaches to enhance the chances of success.

References

1. Stern C, Pertile M, Norris H et al. Chromosome translocations in couples with in-vitro fertilisation implantation failure. *Hum Reprod* 1999; **14**: 2097–101.

2. Levitas E, Lunenfeld E, har-Vardi I et al. Blastocyst-stage embryo transfer in patients who failed to conceive in three or more day 2–3 embryo transfer cycles: a prospective randomized study. *Fertil Steril* 2004; **81**: 567–71.

3. Guerif F, Bidault R, Gasnier O et al. Efficacy of blastocyst transfer after implantation failure. *Reprod Biomed Online* 2004; **9**: 630–6.

4. Das M, Holzer HE. Recurrent implantation failure: gamete and embryo factors. *Fertil Steril Epub* 2012; **97**(5): 1021–7.

5. Simon A, Laufer N. repeated implantation failure: clinical approach. *Fertil Steril* 2012; **97**: 1039–43.

6. Narvekar SA, Gupta N, Shetty N et al. Does local endometrial injury in the nontransfer cycle improve the IVF-ET outcome in the subsequent cycle in patients with previous unsuccessful IVF? A randomized controlled pilot study. *J Hum Reprod Sci* 2010; **3**: 15–19.

7. Potdar N, Gelbaya T, Nardo LG. Endometrial injury to overcome recurrent embryo implantation failure: a systematic review and meta-analysis. *Reprod Biomed Online* 2012; **12**: S1472.

8. Chao K-H, Chen S-U, Chen H-F et al. Assisted hatching increases the implantation and pregnancy rate of in vitro fertilization (IVF)-embryo transfer (ET), but not that of IVF-tubal ET in patients with repeated IVF failures. *Fertil Steril* 1997; **67**: 904–8.

9. Martins WP, Rocha IA, Ferriani RA et al. Assisted hatching of human embryos: a systematic review and meta-analysis of randomized controlled trials. *Hum Reprod Update* 2011; **17**: 438–53.

10. Blockeel C, Schutyser V, De Vos A et al. Prospectively randomized controlled trial of OGS in IVF/ICSI patients with poor implantation. *Reprod Biomed Online* 2008; **17**: 848–54.

11. Urman B, Ata B, Yakin K et al. Luteal phase empirical low molecular weight heparin administration in patients with failed ICSI embryo transfer cycles: a randomized open-labeled pilot trial. *Hum Reprod* 2009; **24**: 1640–7.

Fertility preservation in an adolescent with Turner syndrome

Michel De Vos

General medical, family, and social history

K., the only child of two healthy parents, was diagnosed with Turner syndrome before she was born. An amniocentesis had been performed because of increased nuchal translucency and revealed the presence of 45,XO amniocytes. The pregnancy was uneventful. K. was born at term with a birth weight of 3250 g and a length of 49 cm. After birth, cytogenetic analysis of lymphocytes confirmed 35% 45,XO/65% 46,XX mosaicism. As a baby and a toddler she demonstrated normal neuromotoric development. At the age of 11 months her length was 66.4 cm (<P3) and her weight 8 kg (P3–P25). On examination she had a short neck without webbing and a low hairline. Blood sampling showed low circulating levels of IGF-1. An echocardiogram showed a normal cardiac function. At the age of 2 years, K.'s growth started to deviate from the P3 centile. Growth hormone treatment was initiated when she was aged 4 years. At the age of 9 years she start to develop signs of pubertas praecox, which was probably due to hyperinsulinism secondary to growth hormone treatment and appeared to suggest normal ovarian function. To slow down pubertal development, 425 mg daily of metformin was started. Menarche occurred just before her 12th birthday, at Tanner stage A2 P4 M3. Hormone testing at that stage revealed normal gonadotropin levels and a circulating antimüllerian hormone (AMH) level of 3.77 ng/mL. The endocrinologist referred K. and her parents to a fertility clinic for fertility preservation counseling. Although K. was aware of the diagnosis of Turner syndrome, she had not yet been informed of the consequences for reproduction. At the age of 13 years, at Tanner stage A2 P5 M5, K. had a regular menstruation pattern and clinical examination showed discrete facial acne vulgaris. At the age of 14 years and 4 months, K. measured 152.4 cm. Her BMI was 20.6 kg/m^2. The growth cartilage disks appeared to have closed and growth hormone treatment was therefore discontinued. Metformin was continued at a daily dose of 850 mg.

Referral to the fertility clinic

Soon after K. had been informed by her parents about the increased risk of primary ovarian insufficiency, the family presented at the fertility clinic, where they met a clinical adolescent psychologist and a gynecologist. An in-depth discussion with the family was held with regard to the consequences of Turner syndrome mosaicism on reproductive function and they were counseled about how to cope with the issue of threatening sterility in a 14-year-old.

Fertility investigations

An abdominal ultrasound scan revealed the presence of ovaries of approximately 22 mm by 15 mm and seven antral follicles in each ovary. In view of the genetic condition and its inherent impact on the ovarian follicular pool, K. was offered the opportunity to undergo either ovarian cortex cryopreservation or controlled ovarian stimulation with gonadotropins, followed by oocyte vitrification.

Diagnosis

Adolescent with Turner syndrome mosaicism requesting fertility cryopreservation.

Action plan

Ovarian stimulation was performed using 150 IU rFSH daily in a GnRH antagonist protocol. Follicular development was monitored using regular abdominal ultrasound scans and blood sampling. After 9 days of fixed-dose gonadotropin stimulation, four follicles measuring 18 mm were observed, with another five follicles measuring between 12 and 18 mm. The measured serum estradiol level was 1246 ng/L.

Final oocyte maturation was triggered using 0.2 mg buserelin and transvaginal oocyte retrieval was performed 36 hours later, under general anesthetic. Eight mature oocytes were obtained for closed-straw vitrification. K. had an uneventful recovery.

Outcome

Cryopreservation of eight mature oocytes in an adolescent with Turner syndrome mosaicism. In view of the well-tolerated procedure, K. and her parents have requested the rescheduling of another round of ovarian stimulation and cryopreservation within 3 months from the first oocyte retrieval.

General remarks

With a prevalence of 1 in 2500 female live births, Turner syndrome is the most common sex chromosome abnormality in women. Approximately half of these women have only one X chromosome (monosomy), some have a structural anomaly of an X chromosome, and more than one third have a mosaic form, often with a tissue-specific distribution of cells with a normal karyotype and cells with X chromosome monosomy. Only one third of women with Turner syndrome experience spontaneous pubertal development and primary amenorrhea is common, due to premature and accelerated apoptosis of ovarian follicles. Spontaneous pregnancy is rare and has been reported most commonly in individuals with small X deletions or mosaic Turner syndrome. In the latter, ovarian function is preserved longer although nomograms of ovarian follicular depletion in these individuals have not been established and follicular demise can occur rapidly. In children and adolescents with Turner syndrome, oocyte donation has long been considered the option of first choice, although recent developments in fertility preservation strategies have enhanced the potential for women with Turner syndrome to conceive after fertilization of their own eggs. Hence, it has become fundamental to consider ovarian reserve testing in girls with Turner syndrome to provide them and their families with relevant information concerning fertility and to discuss fertility preservation options. In view of their young age and the delicacy of the topic, it seems appropriate to discuss the subject of fertility preservation in these individuals according to a multidisciplinary approach.

Successful ovarian stimulation followed by oocyte cryopreservation has been described in a 22-year-old woman with Turner syndrome mosaicism (El-Shawarby *et al.* 2010). In some postmenarchal girls with mosaic Turner syndrome, ovarian follicular density as assessed by hormonal and ultrasound ovarian reserve testing appears to offer possibilities for ovarian stimulation. Although ovarian stimulation for oocyte cryopreservation has been described in a premenarchal girl (Reichman *et al.* 2012), it remains to be established whether ovarian response to exogenous gonadotropins in young adolescents and girls at early stages of puberty can be predicted by the same markers of ovarian reserve that are commonly used in adults.

Ovarian cortex cryopreservation, most commonly offered to patients with impending ovarian insufficiency due to gonadotoxic treatment, also merits considering in women with Turner syndrome. Although ovarian cortex allografting has been reported between monozygotic twins who both had 45,XO/46,XX mosaicism, with 23% X monosomy in the donor ovary and 12% X monosomy in the recipient gonad, but discordant ovarian function, resulting in a live birth (Donnez *et al.* 2011), ovarian cryopreservation in these patients is still considered experimental because of uncertainty regarding the dynamics of follicular depletion in these patients, even more so after freezing and thawing. Future prospects for young girls with Turner syndrome include advances in in vitro follicle growth performed on cryopreserved ovarian tissue, although it may be many years before this development becomes routine clinical practice (Telfer and McLaughlin 2011). Nevertheless, important concerns remain: oocytes of women with Turner syndrome have an increased incidence of aneuploidy, and the increased risk of hypertension and preeclampsia in pregnant women with Turner syndrome warrants appropriate counseling and intense antenatal follow-up.

References

Donnez J *et al.* Live birth after allografting of ovarian cortex between monozygotic twins with Turner syndrome (45,XO/46,XX mosaicism) and discordant ovarian function. *Fertil Steril* (2011); **96**(6): 1407–11.

El-Shawarby SA *et al.* Oocyte cryopreservation after controlled ovarian hyperstimulation in mosaic Turner syndrome: another fertility preservation option in a dedicated UK clinic. *BJOG* (2010); **117**(2): 234–7.

Reichman DE *et al.* Fertility preservation using controlled ovarian hyperstimulation and oocyte cryopreservation in a premenarcheal female with myelodysplastic syndrome. *Fertil Steril* (2012); **98**(5): 1225–8.

Telfer EE, McLaughlin M. In vitro development of ovarian follicles. *Semin Reprod Med* (2011); **29**(1): 15–23.

Further reading

Pasquino AM, Passeri F, Pucarelli I, Segni M, Municchi G. Spontaneous pubertal development in Turner's syndrome. Italian Study Group for Turner's Syndrome. *J Clin Endocrinol Metab*. 1997; **82**: 1810–13.

Saenger P, Wikland KA, Conway GS, Davenport M, Gravholt CH, Hintz R *et al.* Fifth International Symposium on Turner Syndrome. Recommendations for the diagnosis and management of Turner syndrome. *J Clin Endocrinol Metab*. 2001; **86**: 3061–9.

A young woman with a low AMH

Christophe Blockeel and Veerle Vloeberghs

Clinical fertility history

A 29-year-old woman with 12 months of infertility presented for investigation. She reported a regular cycle of 27 days and had no history of menorrhagia or dysmenorrhea.

General medical, family, and social history

Her medical history revealed a history of asthma. At the age of 21 years, she was operated for an acute nonperforated appendicitis. The family history was negative. The patient smoked five cigarettes a day.

Examination findings

The patient, who weighed 61 kg and measured 1.65 m (BMI 22 kg/m²), underwent preliminary examinations. The hormonal profile did not show any abnormalities, and an ultrasound scan showed a normal uterus with no ovarian cysts. However, her baseline antral follicle count was only 4. The antimüllerian hormone (AMH) level was 0.54 µg/L.

Her partner's seminal fluid analysis showed a severe oligoasthenoteratozoospermia with no clear cause.

Diagnosis

Both an andrological factor and reduced ovarian reserve were diagnosed, and the couple was advised to undergo IVF treatment with ICSI.

Action plan

Given the expected low response, a higher dose of 300 IU of recombinant FSH was prescribed in a GnRH antagonist protocol. After 8 days of ovarian stimulation, the cycle was cancelled, due to monofollicular growth.

The patient was informed of the poor prognosis for conceiving with further IVF cycles, but a second trial of ovarian stimulation was embarked upon. In the second cycle, a long GnRH agonist protocol was applied, and nasal buserelin (Suprefact) was given for 2 weeks before starting ovarian stimulation with HP-hMG. However, two weeks after the use of the nasal spray, and before the start of ovarian stimulation, a vaginal ultrasound revealed the growth of three large follicles measuring 21, 23, and 25 mm resulting from a presumed flare-up effect. The endometrial thickness was 8 mm. The estradiol level was 728 pg/mL.

At this stage, an injection with hCG 5000 IU was administered for final oocyte maturation and 36 hours later an oocyte retrieval was performed, leading to the pick-up of three mature oocytes. Two were fertilized and developed into embryos of good quality, 8 and 9 blastomeres type 1 and 2 respectively. One embryo was transferred and the other was frozen.

Outcome

Two weeks after the embryo transfer, the pregnancy test was positive, and at 7 weeks of amenorrhea fetal cardiac activity was seen on the ultrasound scan. The patient delivered a healthy baby at term.

General remarks

Besides GnRH antagonists, gonadotropin-releasing hormone agonists (GnRH-a) are still widely used in ovarian stimulation for in vitro fertilization (IVF) treatment to prevent premature LH rise [1]. It is well known that the incidence of functional ovarian cyst development is increased following GnRH-a administration in IVF cycles [2]. Possible explanations include the initial transient flare-up effect of the GnRH agonist on gonadotropins [3].

This flare-up response can be excessive, and several case reports have described the occurrence of ovarian hyperstimulation syndrome following the administration of just one dose of GnRH agonist [4, 5, 6]. The mechanism of the elevation of FSH and LH above the threshold for allowing follicular growth remains unclear. However, it has been suggested that desensitization of hypothalamic pituitary GnRH receptors blocks the negative feedback effect of elevated estradiol and that there may be an augmented effect of FSH and LH on the ovary. Pregnancy following this therapy is extremely rare and has been reported only once [7].

In this case, a pragmatic approach to the observed flare response was adopted, as it was considered unlikely that a better result would arise in a further stimulated cycle.

References

1. Macklon NS, Stouffer RL, Giudice LC, Fauser BC. The science behind 25 years of ovarian stimulation for in vitro fertilization. *Endocr Rev* 2006; **27**(2): 170–207.

2. Tarlatzis BC, Fauser BC, Kolibianakis EM, Diedrich K, Rombauts L, Devroey P. GnRH antagonists in ovarian stimulation for IVF. *Hum Reprod Update* 2006; **12**(4): 333–40.

3. Feldburg D, Ashkenazi J, Dicker D, Yeshaya A, Goldman GA, Goldman JA. Ovarian cyst formation: a complication of gonadotropin-releasing hormone agonist therapy. *Fertil Steril* 1989; **51**: 42–4.

4. Yeh J, Barbieri RL, Ravnikar VA. Ovarian hyperstimulation associated with the sole use of leuprolide for ovarian suppression. *J In Vitro Fert Embryo Transf* 1989; **6**(4): 261–3.

5. Weissman A, Barash A, Shapiro H, Casper RF. Ovarian hyperstimulation following the sole administration of agonistic analogues of gonadotrophin releasing hormone. *Hum Reprod* 1998; **13**(12): 3421–4.

6. Qublan HS, Beni-Merei Z, Megdadi M, Al-Quraan G. Ovarian hyperstimulation syndrome following the sole administration of injectable gonadotropin-releasing hormone agonist (triptorelin) for the pituitary down-regulation and in vitro fertilization treatment: report of two cases. *Arch Gynecol Obstet* 2009; **279**(2): 221–3.

7. Azem F, Almog B, Ben-Yosef D, Kapustiansky R, Wagman I, Amit A. First live birth following IVF-embryo transfer and use of GnRHa alone for ovarian stimulation. *Reprod Biomed Online* 2009; **19**(2): 162–4.

The patient who bleeds in the early luteal phase

Robert Lahoud and Manveen (Manny) Mangat

Case history

C.H. presented at the age of 33 years with a 2-year history of secondary infertility. She was of South-East Asian descent and had had a termination of pregnancy in 1993 for social reasons. At the time of presentation, she reported irregular menstrual cycles (normal flow) ranging between 33 and 42 days in cycle length. She had no hirsutism or acne. The patient denied any dysmenorrhea or dyspareunia, but did describe a small amount of premenstrual spotting. Her weight was 54 kg and her height was 163 cm giving a BMI of 20.3 kg/m².

C.H. had no significant past medical or surgical history. She was a nonsmoker and had a family history of diabetes mellitus. Physical and gynecological examination was unremarkable.

Investigations

Ultrasound showed a normal-appearing retroverted uterus with a small subserous fibroid. The ovaries were not described as polycystic. The fallopian tubes were patent and the uterine cavity appeared normal.

The day 2 FSH was 5 IU/L and the LH was 3 IU/L, within the normal range for her age. Thyroid function tests and prolactin levels were normal. There was no documented ovulation when progesterone levels were measured.

The patient's husband was 36 years old. He had a past history of an orchidopexy following testicular torsion. He also suffered from depression and was treated with an SSRI He blamed his ejaculatory dysfunction and decreased libido on his medications. He was also being treated for hypertension with an angiotensin II receptor antagonist.

He had two semen analyses, showing oligoasthenozoospermia. The hormone profile was normal with FSH 3.4 IU/L, testosterone 19 nmol/L, prolactin 90 mU/L, and TSH 0.76 mU/L.

A scrotal ultrasound was reported as normal.

Diagnosis

1. Male factor infertility
2. Ovulatory dysfunction

Treatment

The couple progressed to IVF/ICSI treatment. Table 22.1 summarizes the treatment cycles and outcomes.

Table 22.1 Summary of treatment cycles and outcomes.

Cycle no. and type	No. of oocytes collected	No. and quality of embryos transferred	Luteal support	Cycle outcome	Comment
1st LDR	16	1 Bl-A gr	Cr 90/d	Early bleed not pregnant	
2nd LDR	16	1 eBl-A gr	Cr 90/d	Early bleed not pregnant	
3rd Antag	7	1 Bl-A gr (2 frozen Bl)	Cr 90/d	Early bleed not pregnant	
FET 1/2			Prog. 200 mg bd	Cancelled – spot bleeding	
FET 3		1 Bl (1 did not thaw)	Prog. 200 mg bd	Not pregnant	
4th Antag.	7	1 Bl-A gr	Prog. 200 mg/day	Early bleed not pregnant	Progesterone test 89 pmol/L 7 days post oocyte pick-up
5th Antag.	13	1 Bl-A gr	Prog. 200 mg bd	Early bleed not pregnant	LH (Luveris) 75 IU from day 6
6th Antag.	16	1 Bl-A gr	Prog. 200 mg bd	Early bleed but hCG test 55, progesterone 10 (low)	LMW heparin given
7th Antag.	8	2 Bl-A gr	Prog. 200 mg bd and hCG 5000 IUX1	Pregnant: Live birth female 3300 g	

LDR, long down regulation protocol; Antag., antagonist protocol; B, blastocyst; eBl, early blastocyst; A gr, A grade; Cr 90/d, Crinone gel 90 mg/day; Prog., progesterone pessaries; hCG, human chorionic gonadotropin/Pregnyl; LMW heparin, low-molecular-weight heparin/enaxoparin sodium/Clexane 20 mg/day.

Case review

- C.H. was at risk of ovarian hyperstimulation syndrome (OHSS) as noted by elevated estradiol levels. As a result, progesterone instead of hCG was used for luteal support. With each of the cycles vaginal bleeding started before the planned pregnancy test (16 days post oocyte retrieval).
- To deal with the luteal defect, increased doses of progesterone and finally the addition of hCG resulted in a successful pregnancy.
- The embryo quality was possibly affected by high levels of sperm DNA fragmentation. For a patient in her early thirties very few embryos were suitable for cryopreservation.
- Further investigations were performed following the third cycle:
  - **C.H.:** Normal karyotype 46,XX, normal autoimmune and thrombophilia screens.
  - A hysteroscopy showed normal endometrium. The laparoscopy revealed mild endometriosis, which was treated. She also had a 2-cm subserous fibroid of no clinical significance.

- **Husband:** Normal karyotype, TUNEL assay (sperm DNA fragmentation) 27% (moderate fragmentation).

- To improve the chance of implantation, laser-assisted hatching and heparin injection were used empirically. The patient was also undergoing acupuncture treatment utilizing an external Chinese herbalist. All of these therapies are controversial and it is unclear whether they made a difference.

C.H. has returned for three further stimulated and two frozen cycles. Again the same protocol of increased luteal support was used. Even in the unsuccessful cycles, the bleeding occurred much closer to and even after the pregnancy test day (16 days post oocyte retrieval). With the 10th stimulated cycle another successful pregnancy was achieved. This time a live male infant weighing 3800 g was delivered at term. No fetal anomalies were recorded.

In summary, over 4 years and following 10 stimulated IVF/ICSI cycles, C.H. and her partner finally achieved their aim of a family. Looking back at the issues causing recurrent implantation failure, the overall picture is a complex one. It does appear, though, that C.H. displayed a tendency toward early bleeding in the luteal phase. This occurred both in fresh and hormone-assisted frozen cycles. The most likely reason for the early bleeding is progesterone deficiency. Absorption of vaginal progesterone preparations can vary between individuals. An individualized approach as in this case appears reasonable.

This case has led to significant changes in the management of the luteal phase in my practice. In any patient identified as bleeding early in the luteal phase despite luteal support, progesterone supplementation is increased and the use of hCG is considered in a subsequent cycle. Serum progesterone testing is done on days 5 and 10 following oocyte retrieval. The addition of oral estradiol may be considered.

That said, the debate continues about whether increased intervention in the luteal phase is effective.

Discussion

The luteal phase is defined as the period between ovulation and either the establishment of pregnancy or the onset of menstruation usually 2 weeks after.

From the first attempts at IVF in the late 1970s, it was clear that luteal phase disruption posed a potential cause for an unsuccessful IVF cycle. The luteal phase has been extensively studied in ART cycles, resulting in an undisputed need for luteal phase support following controlled ovarian stimulation.

The use of GnRH agonists and antagonists causes disruption via prolonged suppression of LH secretion and premature luteolysis respectively. It is also postulated that the supraphysiological hormone levels during controlled ovarian stimulation cause negative feedback on LH pulsatility, thereby rendering the corpus luteum dysfunctional [1].

The importance of progesterone for maintaining early pregnancy has long been established [2].

More recent studies using GnRH agonist triggers for antagonist cycles also show that even though the LH surge amplitude is comparable, the duration is shortened to only 24–48 hours versus 8 days, if triggering with hCG. This has been shown to cause a sudden drop in hormones, leading to a luteolytic effect, shorter luteal phase with earlier bleeding, and lower pregnancy rates.

A recent Cochrane review published in 2011 reevaluated the data, confirming that progesterone (synthetic over micronized), largely irrespective of the route of administration, was the most effective and safest option for luteal phase support, further supporting the argument that increased luteal support may not be beneficial.

A short summary of different types of luteal phase support

- *hCG:*
    - Good luteal support.
    - No difference in pregnancy rates when compared to progesterone.
    - Increased risk of OHSS.
- *hCG and progesterone:*
    - No additional benefit seen but may reduce luteal bleeding due to drop in estradiol.
- *Progesterone:*
    - **Intramuscular (IM):** as effective as hCG, no increased risk of OHSS but painful to inject (as given in oil vehicle) and can cause allergic reactions and occasional sterile abscess formation. Only one meta-analysis [3] showed IM progesterone to have increased clinical pregnancy and delivery rates over vaginal preparations.
    - **Oral:** subject to first-pass hepatic metabolism, therefore high doses are required that will produce sedation. Micronization improves absorption and bioavailability.
    - **Vaginal:** as effective as IM in all studies but one. Targeted delivery. Wide application as first choice due to ease of use, patient comfort and effectiveness. May be given as gel or pessaries.
- *Progesterone and estrogen:*
    - Earlier small heterogeneous studies have shown possible benefit with addition of transdermal estrogen.
    - No added benefit in more recent reviews [3].
- *GnRH agonists, either alone or in addition to progesterone:*
    - Recent novel luteal phase support that may act on the pituitary gonadotrophs, the endometrium, and the embryo itself through locally expressed GnRH receptors [4]. It has been shown to enhance pregnancy rates in both agonist and antagonist protocols, but it is too early to adopt across the board and further large prospective trials are needed.

Timing and duration

- If progesterone is commenced too early it is not beneficial to the endometrium.
- hCG trigger covers the patient for 5–8 days.
- Recent studies have shown no difference in pregnancy and miscarriage rates if luteal support was ceased with positive pregnancy test (12–14 days after transfer) versus continuing to 7 weeks.

Should progesterone be measured in the luteal phase?

A reliable diagnostic tool for adequate luteal support is still elusive as serum progesterone level is not always reflective of the endometrial status. Also there is wide daily variation in the progesterone levels, making reliable interpretation of progesterone results difficult.

Frozen embryo transfer cycles (FET)

In anovulatory patients hormone replacement treatment (HRT) cycles have been preferred. Down regulated HRT cycles appear more successful than nondown regulated cycles. The addition of GnRH agonist down regulation as well as HRT increases the complexity of the cycle, as well as the time taken to complete the cycle. Based on a recent Swedish randomized controlled trial [5], the addition of luteal progesterone in natural FETs may be considered beneficial.

Investigating abnormal uterine bleeding

It is important to investigate abnormal uterine bleeding thoroughly. In this case the original normal Hycosy ultrasound was followed up by a hysteroscopy, endometrial biopsy, and laparoscopy. The endometriosis detected was treated at laparoscopy. Most abnormal bleeding in IVF cycles is likely to be hormonal, but endometrial polyps and endometriosis are other common causes. Understandably, endometrial malignancy and endometritis need to be excluded.

Final comments

The case of C.H. is obviously a complex one, having resulted in two successful live births. The question remains unanswered whether the increase in luteal support or the other interventions resulted in success. The argument will continue about what type of luteal support and at what dose. In the case of early bleeding, increased intervention is warranted as it is unlikely to be harmful and will at least give the appearance that "all that is possible has been done."

References

1. Sonntag B, Ludwig M. An integrated view on the luteal phase: diagnosis and treatment in subfertility. *Clinical Endocrinology* 2012; 77(4): 500–7.

2. Pritts EA, Atwood AK. Luteal phase support in infertility treatment: a meta-analysis of the randomized trials. *Human Reproduction* 2002; 17(9): 2287–99.

3. Kolibianakis EM, Venetis CA, Papanikolaou EG, Diedrich K, Tarlatzis BC, Griesinger G. Estrogen addition to progesterone for luteal phase support in cycles stimulated with GnRH analogues and gonadotrophins for IVF: a systematic review and meta-analysis. *Human Reproduction* 2008; 23(6): 1346–54.

4. Tesarik J, Hazout A, Mendoza-Tesarik R, Mendoza N, Mendoza C. Beneficial effect of luteal-phase GnRH agonist administration on embryo implantation after ICSI in both GnRH agonist- and antagonist-treated ovarian stimulation cycles. *Human Reproduction* 2006; 21(10): 2572–9.

5. Bjuresten K, Landgren B-M, Hovatta O, Stavreus-Evers A. Luteal phase progesterone increases live birth rate after frozen embryo transfer. *Fertility and Sterility* 2011; 95(2): 534–7.

Threatened OHSS in a long GnRH agonist protocol

E. Papanikolaou

Clinical fertility history

A 27-year-old woman presented with primary infertility of 5 years' duration and of male origin. She was already under stimulation with 150 IU of HMG in a GnRH agonist protocol for IVF and experiencing already high ovarian response. She had a history of two previous IVF trials, both of them complicated with severe OHSS. For this reason she requested a second opinion as to whether to stop or continue the stimulation. None of the previous IVF cycles had been successful.

General medical, family, and social history

Her medical history was unremarkable and she was not a smoker.

Examination findings

Physical examination recorded a weight of 69 kg and height of 160 cm. Gynecological examination was impossible due to abdominal and pelvic discomfort.

Fertility investigations

Previous investigations indicated a history of polycystic ovaries with ovulatory cycles. Tubal patency testing was normal. Sperm analysis indicated severe oligoasthenospermia with fewer than 1 million sperm and less than 10% motility.

Other clinical investigations

The transvaginal ultrasound revealed more than 10 medium follicles (11–12 mm) in each ovary, and a small amount of fluid already present in the pouch of Douglas. The estradiol level was greater than 3000 pg/mL.

Diagnosis

The patient was at high risk for developing OHSS.

Action plan

After consulting the couple, it was decided to continue the stimulation and to freeze all produced zygotes. Prednisolone 10 mg/day was initiated, and the gonadotropin dose was decreased to 100 IU/day. Three days later, more than three follicles of 17 mm were observed on ultrasound scan, and so final oocyte maturation was triggered with 5000 IU of hCG. The estradiol level was now 7500 pg/mL and that of progesterone was 1.4 ng/mL. Twenty-seven oocytes were retrieved of which 20 were considered mature. Ten oocytes were fertilized and seven top-quality day-3 embryos were cryopreserved. Cabergoline 0.25 mg was also administered for 5 days. The patient developed symptoms consistent with moderate early OHSS without any need for hospitalization and from day 8 in the luteal phase her physical activity returned to normal.

Outcome

After her second spontaneous menstruation following completion of the stimulated IVF cycle, an estrogen substitution cycle was commenced and two thawed embryos were transferred. She had a singleton pregnancy and a healthy boy was born 9 months later.

General remarks

The first wrong decision regarding this patient was to treat her with a long GnRH agonist protocol. The protocol of choice for high-responders, especially with a history of OHSS, is the antagonist protocol [1]. Apart from lower incidence of OHSS, there is also the option to replace hCG triggering with agonist triggering whereby OHSS is almost completely eliminated [2]. Unfortunately, during the long protocol this alternative does not exist; there are other modalities, however, that should be applied. The first is to lower the gonadotropin dose. The second is to trigger with reduced hCG dose, 5000 or even 3500 IU. The third is to cancel the embryo transfer and to vitrify all embryos. In that case, a well-established cryopreservation program is required. If the clinical condition of the patient allows, the transfer a single blastocyst can be considered, with concomitant administration of medications that have been shown to reduce the risk of OHSS such as cortisol, and dopamine agonists should be applied [3]. Therefore, even in the context of treatment with the long GnRH agonist protocol, modifications to reduce the incidence of OHSS are available. However, prevention is the keystone of contemporary treatment. Low-dose gonadotropin guided by markers of ovarian reserve such as AMH levels constitutes the first-line approach [4].

References

1. Humaidan P, Quartarolo J, Papanikolaou EG. Preventing ovarian hyperstimulation syndrome: guidance for the clinician. *Fertil Steril* 2010; **94**: 389–400.

2. Humaidan P, Kol S, Papanikolaou EG; Copenhagen GnRH Agonist Triggering Workshop Group. GnRH agonist for triggering of final oocyte maturation: time for a change of practice? *Hum Reprod Update* 2011; **17**: 510–24.

3. Shaltout A, Shohyab A, Youssef MA. Can dopamine agonist at a low dose reduce ovarian hyperstimulation syndrome in women at risk undergoing ICSI treatment cycles? A randomized controlled study. *Eur J Obstet Gynecol Reprod Biol* 2012; **165**(2): 254–8.

4. Papanikolaou EG, Humaidan P, Polyzos N, Kalantaridou S, Kol S, Benadiva C, Tournaye H, Tarlatzis B. New algorithm for OHSS prevention. *Reprod Biol Endocrinol* 2011; **9**: 147.

An endometrial polyp detected during ovarian stimulation for IVF

Human M. Fatemi and Biljana Popovic Todorovic

Clinical fertility history

A 22-year-old white woman patient with a primary infertility for 3 years was seen at the outpatient clinic. Prior her visit, the patient had undergone six intrauterine insemination cycles and three IVF cycles with an embryo transfer in another center. Unfortunately, pregnancy was not achieved. The etiology of infertility was due to oligoasthenoteratospermia of her partner. The patient had no previous medical, gynecological, or surgical history. The patient had a family history of diabetes and arterial hypertension. Her body mass index was 33 kg/m². A pelvic examination revealed normal external genitalia; Pap smear was obtained without any difficulties. Bimanual examination revealed no pelvic tenderness or masses and a normal uterus size.

Fertility investigation

As a part of routine examination, an ultrasound was performed on day 3 of the cycle, which revealed an antral follicle count of 6 on the right ovary and 7 on the left ovary. A normal uterus was visualized. No intracavitary abnormalities could be visualized. Serum hormone levels of FSH, LH, estradiol, progesterone, and prolactin were all within the normal range. The husband's sperm parameters were reported as follows: concentration 11 million/mL, motility A+B 27%, and morphology according to the strict criteria of Kruger was 3% normal. A diagnosis of primary infertility due to the male factor was confirmed and the decision was taken to start IVF-ICSI treatment.

Ovarian stimulation, IVF-ICSI procedures

RecFSH was initiated in the afternoon of the second day of the cycle at a dose of 200 IU/day. The dose of recFSH remained unchanged until day 5 of stimulation. To inhibit premature LH rise, it was planned to administer GnRH 0.25 mL from the morning of day 6 of stimulation. On day 6 of stimulation the patient was seen with a request for ultrasound and endocrine assessment. However, ultrasound showed the presence of an intracavitary polyp 9 × 8 mm in dimension, disturbing the endometrial triple line. The findings were explained clearly to the patient and her husband and all the possibilities were discussed. Following consideration of published evidence suggesting that polyp resection can be safely performed without cycle cancellation, it was decided to resect the polyp just prior to oocyte retrieval. GnRH antagonist was initiated on day 6 and recFSH was continued. On day 7 of stimulation with three leading follicles of 14 mm, the patient underwent a hysteroscopic resection of the polyp. The procedure was carried out under mild sedation using a 5-mm diameter continuous-flow hysteroscope with 30° direction of view (Olympus NV, Aartselaar, Belgium).

Normal saline solution was used for the distention of the uterine cavity at a pressure of 20–50 mmHg. During the procedure no cervical dilatation was used. During the assessment of the uterine cavity an anterior polyp of approximately 9 mm diameter was visualized and was removed using scissors and grasping forceps. After the intervention and removal of the polyp, a second look was performed to confirm that the polyp had been removed completely. By reducing the pressure during the second look, possible bleeding from the site of the resected polyp was prevented. Two hours after the procedure the patient was able to leave the hospital. On days 8 and 9, the stimulation with recFSH and GnRH antagonist was continued and the patient was triggered with 10 000 IU of hCG given subcutaneously for final oocyte maturation; 36 hours later, under local anesthesia, egg retrieval was conducted. Twelve cumulus–oocyte complexes (COCs) were retrieved with 10 MII oocytes, eight fertilized with ICSI, and on day 5 one embryo was transferred and three blastocysts were frozen. As luteal phase support, natural micronized progesterone 400 mg twice daily was administered vaginally. Two weeks later a serum hCG test was positive. At 7 weeks the patient had a singleton ongoing pregnancy with a positive heartbeat.

Discussion

In human reproduction there are two main factors which are crucial for a successful pregnancy: one is the embryo quality and the other is endometrial receptivity [1].

There is still no consensus regarding the impact on implantation of polyps or other minor malformations in the uterine cavity [2]. A variety of retrospective trials have been conducted which demonstrated a negative impact of minor uterine abnormalities. However, there is a lack of prospective randomized trials. Endometrial polyps have been diagnosed in 1.4% of patients undergoing IVF treatment [3]. A trial published recently by Fatemi *et al.* [2] failed to demonstrate any impact of minor uterine abnormalities detected during office hysteroscopy on the impact on IVF, mainly due to the limited number of patients. Moreover, it seems to be difficult to include patients in such a trial.

Hysteroscopic polypectomy during stimulation cycles might damage the endometrium; however, several studies have demonstrated that endometrial manipulation such as biopsy [4] or polypectomy has no impact on embryo implantation. Moreover, it seems that hysteroscopy and endometrial biopsy even increase the chance of implantation [5]. While the underlying mechanism is unknown, it has been proposed that endometrial sampling or injury might increase endometrial receptivity by inducing a healing response. During this process there is a massive secretion of a range of cytokines and growth factors which are also known to be involved in implantation [6]. However, there is still insufficient evidence to support injuring the endometrium as a routine procedure.

Moreover, there is ongoing debate regarding the size of polyps that should be resected. Lass *et al.* [3] demonstrated in a retrospective trial that polyps less than 2 cm should not be resected. However, there is still a lack of clear randomized control studies to demonstrate this. In the present case, hysteroscopic polyp resection during the follicular phase of an IVF cycle appeared not to have a negative impact on implantation and ongoing pregnancy.

However, since this is a case report, one cannot draw a definite conclusion. Further prospective randomized trials are needed to confirm the safety of hysteroscopic polypectomy during stimulation. Moreover, proper randomized controlled trials should be conducted to evaluate whether systematic, atraumatic, diagnostic hysteroscopy should be performed in all patients undergoing IVF to improve endometrial receptivity due to stimulation and/or reaction of the endometrium.

References

1. Norwitz ER, Schust DJ. Fisher SJ. Implantation and the survival of early pregnancy. *N Engl J Med* 2001; **8**(345): 1400–8.

2. Fatemi HM, Kasius JC, Timmermans A *et al.* Prevalence of unsuspected uterine cavity abnormalities diagnosed by office hysteroscopy prior to in vitro fertilization. *Hum Reprod* 2010; **25**: 1959–65.

3. Lass A, Williams G, Abusheikha N *et al.* The effect of endometrial polyps on outcomes of in vitro fertilization (IVF) cycles. *J Assist Reprod Genet* 1999; **16**: 410–15.

4. van der Gaast MH, Beier-Hellwig K, Fauser BC *et al.* Endometrial secretion aspiration prior to embryo transfer does not reduce implantation rates. *Reprod Biomed Online* 2003; **7**: 105–9.

5. Batioglu S, Kaymak O. Does hysteroscopic polypectomy without cycle cancellation affect IVF? *Reprod Biomed Online* 2005; **10**: 767–9.

6. Basak S, Dubanchet S, Zourbas S *et al.* Expression of pro-inflammatory cytokines in mouse blastocysts during implantation: modulation by steroid hormones. *Am J Reprod Immunol* 2002; **47**: 2–11.

Fluid in the endometrial cavity during IVF treatment

Carolien M. Boomsma and Nick S. Macklon

Clinical fertility history

A 36-year-old woman presented with secondary infertility and secondary amenorrhea and previously diagnosed polycystic ovary syndrome. There were no complaints of dysfunctional blood loss, hirsutism, acne, or other endocrinological symptoms. After failed ovulation induction with clomiphene citrate and gonadotropins, she had conceived after IVF treatment and delivered a healthy son by primary cesarean section because of a placenta praevia totalis. The cesarean section was complicated by excessive blood loss of 2000 mL. After the cesarean section she developed sepsis, the cause of which was uncertain. She was treated for presumed mastitis; however, endometritis, intra-abdominal postoperative infection, or urosepsis were not excluded.

General medical, family, and social history

These provide no information of interest.

Examination findings

BMI 19 kg/m^2 (height 1.67 m, weight 51 kg). Blood pressure 135/85 mmHg.

Fertility investigations

Gynecological investigation showed no abnormalities. On ultrasound examination a normal aspect of the uterus was seen with polycystic ovaries, and no hydrosalpinges. Previous fertility investigation showed a normal hysterosalpingogram. Laboratory investigation showed a normal level of estrogen and gonadotropins (estradiol 250 pmol/L, FSH 6.3 IU/L, LH 5.9 IU/L, and progesterone 3.6 nmol/L). Further endocrinological investigation showed no evidence of hyperandrogenism or signs of a Sheehan syndrome (despite the substantial blood loss at previous operative delivery). Semen analysis revealed normal results.

Diagnosis and action plan

The diagnosis polycystic of ovary syndrome (PCOS) was made based on amenorrhea and polycystic ovaries (Rotterdam criteria). After her previous IVF treatment eight embryos had been cryopreserved. A frozen–thaw transfer in an artificial cycle was planned.

Course of treatment

Following down regulation with GnRH agonist treatment, the endometrium was primed by administering oral estradiol 4 mg daily. However, after 17 days of priming the patient reported daily persistent spotting of blood despite elevation of the dose of estradiol to 8 mg per day. On ultrasound investigation the endometrium was thin and 4 mm fluid in the endometrial cavity was seen. These symptoms and signs in, combination with her history of a complicated cesarean section with postoperative sepsis, were suggestive of Asherman syndrome (intrauterine adhesions). A hysteroscopy was performed. In the cervical channel filmy adhesions were seen, which were removed by perforation with the scope. In the endometrial cavity no abnormalities were seen: no adhesions, no signs of inflammation, and no endometrial cavity niche due to cesarean section.

After a progesterone-induced withdrawal bleed, a second cycle of estradiol priming using 6 mg/day was started without GnRH down regulation. Persistent bleeding in combination with a thin endometrium with fluid on ultrasound investigation occurred and the cycle was cancelled.

A further attempt to prime the endometrium using 8 mg/day oral estradiol was undertaken after a progesterone-induced withdrawal bleeding. Once again, the cycle was complicated by persistent blood loss in combination with fluid (possibly blood) in the endometrial cavity, after which transdermal estradiol was added (1×/3 days bandage estradiol 100 µg/24 h). The clinical picture was unchanged thereafter. Progesterone (Provera) was started thereafter and due to ongoing blood loss a microcurettage was performed after 8 days of combined progesterone–estradiol treatment for endometrial histological dating and to exclude malignancy. Histology showed secretory changes of the epithelial compartment fitting cycle day 22, although the stromal cells were a few days behind. No signs of inflammation or malignancy were reported.

A fourth artificial cycle was started with a high dose of estradiol both oral and transdermal. Due to persistent intrauterine fluid accumulation, the fluid was aspirated from the endometrial cavity with an embryo transfer catheter and progesterone was started (2 × 2/day vaginal Utrogestan 100 mg). An embryo transfer was planned thereafter, but the endometrial fluid recurred and the cycle was cancelled.

Subsequently, endometrial priming was planned by ovulation induction with gonadotropins (recombinant FSH). After stimulation with 50 IU recFSH blood loss returned and the dose was raised to 100 IU/day. The cycle was cancelled due to aggravation of blood loss and persistent thin endometrium, despite normal follicular growth and normal rising estradiol levels but notable low LH levels (<0.5 IU/L). A new cycle was started with 125 IU urinary FSH containing some LH activity. During this cycle, blood loss and ultrasonic intrauterine fluid disappeared after multifollicular growth was achieved with estradiol levels up to 2566 pmol/L and endometrial thickness of 6 mm. Two cryopreserved embryos were successfully transferred. The patient received three doses of subcutaneous hCG 5000 IU for luteal support. Shortly after, she was admitted to the hospital with a mild ovarian hyperstimulation syndrome with a considerable amount of peritoneal free fluid and enlarged ovaries on vaginal ultrasound investigation. There were no signs of infection. She achieved pregnancy, but unfortunately this ended in a spontaneous abortion in the first trimester.

Again, a cycle with 75 IU urinary FSH and LH was started. After monofollicular growth to 16 mm, bleeding stopped and on ultrasound the endometrium measured 10 mm and no fluid was observed within the cavity. hCG 5000 IU was given. However, shortly after the patient reported substantial blood loss and an endometrial thickness of 3 mm was seen. The cycle was cancelled again.

A subsequent cycle was started with urinary FSH after down regulation with a GnRH agonist begun on day 21 of the previous cycle. Again because of substantial blood loss the cycle was cancelled and restarted in a similar manner. In order to exclude her own menstrual cycle from interfering, a natural cycle was awaited before mild ovarian stimulation was restarted. After a spontaneous menstruation, 112.5 IU urinary FSH was started and raised to 150 IU. Multifollicular growth was obtained with disappearance of endometrial fluid. After hCG injection, two cryoembryos were transferred and she conceived. No luteal support was given.

Outcome

The patient achieved a healthy live birth. She delivered at term by uncomplicated cesarean section.

General remarks

In total it took one year and a half for this patient to conceive from the already available cryopreserved embryos with one miscarriage in the meantime. The difficult treatment pathway caused considerable stress for this couple, but was ultimately successful. The underlying differential diagnosis included Asherman syndrome, hydrosalpinges/tubal infertility, endometritis or endometrial malignancy, endometrial fluid accumulation, and lastly loss from a niche resulting from previous cesarean section. However, no signs of these were found on previous hysterosalpingography, hysteroscopy, and histology examination. In conclusion, dysfunctional voiding as an exclusion diagnosis was made.

In a large retrospective study, intrauterine fluid accumulation >4 mm observed on the day of oocyte retrieval has been reported to be detrimental to IVF outcome [1]. Clinical data of 1557 infertility patients undergoing IVF were analyzed, showing an incidence of endometrial fluid accumulation of 3%. Tubal infertility rather than the presence of hydrosalpinges was associated with the presence of endometrial fluid. Forty-six patients with endometrial cavity fluid were compared to a control group of 134 patients with a bilateral salpingectomy without endometrial cavity fluid. No significant difference was found in clinical pregnancy rate between the patients with fluid <3.5 mm (which usually disappeared at the time of embryo transfer) and the control group (36% versus 30% respectively). In women with a fluid accumulation >3.5 mm at ultrasonography, no pregnancies occurred.

There is substantial evidence that endometrial cavity fluid due to the presence of a hydrosalpinx is detrimental to embryo implantation; possibly by embryotoxic factors, a lack of nutrients, and interference with the embryonic–endometrial interaction. A Cochrane meta-analysis including five RCTs involving 646 women concluded that surgical treatment prior to IVF of women with hydrosalpinges compared to no intervention was associated with a significant increase in clinical pregnancy rates (Peto OR 2.31, 95% CI 1.48 to 3.62 for laparoscopic salpingectomy; Peto OR 4.66, 95% CI 2.47 to 10.01 for laparoscopic occlusion of fallopian tubes) [2]. Comparison of tubal occlusion to salpingectomy did not show a significant advantage of either surgical procedure. Different studies have concluded that placement of Essure micro inserts is an effective method of proximal tubal occlusion of the hydrosalpinx with good outcome after IVF; however, no RCTs have yet been performed [2].

PCOS has also been associated with the development of endometrial cavity fluid. Over-reactive fluid secretion by the genital tract during ART as a result of supraphysiological estrogen levels has been proposed as a mechanism in the development of endometrial fluid accumulation [3;4].

IVF outcomes in 24 infertility patients with PCOS and 14 with tubal factor infertility in whom endometrial fluid was detected were compared to 94 women with PCOS and 160 women with tubal pathology in whom no sonographic abnormalities were seen [3]. When endometrial fluid persisted until the day of embryo transfer, the procedure was cancelled and the patients were excluded from the study. No differences in pregnancy rates were seen in women with PCOS with or without fluid accumulation. The authors conclude that when fluid collection inside the endometrial cavity is first seen during ovarian stimulation of women with PCOS undergoing IVF, embryo transfer can be performed safely if the fluid has disappeared and not returned by the day of embryo transfer [3].

Treatment options with endometrial cavity fluid during ovarian stimulation in ART include expectant treatment, postponing embryo transfer with cryopreservation of the embryos, transvaginal sonographically guided fluid aspiration, and other subsidiary modifications and optimizations in ART [4]. Expectant treatment is particularly appropriate for women without tubal infertility. Akman et al. showed that in 89% of women with PCOS with sonographic fluid accumulation, fluid appeared early during ovarian stimulation or after hCG administration and disappeared at the time of embryo transfer [3]. Modifications to ovarian stimulation protocols may include application of mild ovarian stimulation and a modified natural cycle [4]. In the present case, in the artificial cycle after estradiol priming of the endometrium, progesterone was provided for endometrial stabilization. This was not successful, however. Thereafter, since regular therapy of endometrial preparation by an artificial cycle did not succeed, priming by stimulation with gonadotropins was attempted. With this regimen, fluid in the endometrial cavity indeed disappeared after (multi)follicular growth rather than high-dose estradiol priming in an artificial cycle. Transvaginal sonographically guided fluid aspiration was attempted since excessive fluid accumulation in women without tubal infertility has been shown to be usually reactive, self-limiting, and seldom recurrent in the same cycle [4].

In conclusion, endometrial cavity fluid during ART is a challenging problem for the clinician. It has been argued that endometrial cavity fluid accumulation observed in patients with PCOS may represent a different clinical entity from that in patients with tubal disease [3, 4]. Endometrial cavity fluid accumulation during ovarian stimulation impairs the ART outcome in women with tubal factor infertility, but not in PCOS where endometrial fluid accumulation was generated physiologically or reactively during ART. The presented case is somewhat different from those presented in the literature, since there was continuous vaginal blood loss next to fluid (blood) accumulation in utero. Since evidence based medicine does not help us in cases like these, we had to rely on empirical "trial and error." Treatment of endometrial cavity fluid during ART should be individualized according to the cause, the stage of appearance, and the amount of accumulation [3].

References

1. He RH, Gao HJ, Li YQ et al. The associated factors to endometrial cavity fluid and the relevant impact on the IVF-ET outcome. *Reprod Biol Endocrinol* 2010; 8: 46.

2. Johnson N, van Voorst S, Sowter MC et al. Surgical treatment for tubal disease in women due to undergo in vitro fertilisation. *Cochrane Database Syst Rev* 2010; (1): CD002125. DOI: 10.1002/14651858.

3.   Akman MA, Erden HF, Bahceci M. Endometrial fluid visualized through ultrasonography during ovarian stimulation in IVF cycles impairs the outcome in tubal factor, but not PCOS, patients. *Hum Reprod* 2005; **20**: 906–9.

4.   He RH, Zhua XM. How to deal with fluid in the endometrial cavity during assisted reproductive techniques. *Curr Opin Obstet Gynecol* 2011; **23**: 190–4.

Chapter

26

Tubal embryo transfer

A novel approach to managing difficult uterine access

Andrew Murray and John Hutton

Clinical fertility history

A 34-year-old woman presented with amenorrhea for 18 months after a previous cone biopsy in 2002 for persistent abnormal cervical cytology. She had previously had a pregnancy termination, a lower-segment cesarean section, and two large loop excisions of transformation zone (LLETZ) procedures.

General medical, family, and social history

The patient was otherwise fit and well but had recently separated and was seeking treatment as a single woman.

Examination findings

On examination, there was no identifiable cervix.

Fertility investigations

Transvaginal ultrasound measured the residual cervical tissue length as 0.5–2.0 cm; the uterine cavity was distended by a 3-cm hematometra.

Diagnosis

Severe cervical stenosis with coexisiting potential for cervical incompetence and associated increased risk of preterm labor.

Action plan

Menstruation was suppressed with continuous combined oral contraceptive therapy, and after 3 months, the hematometra resolved.

A laparoscopic cervical cerclage was undertaken using 5-mm Mersilene tape (Ethicon). Pregnancy was subsequently postponed, but the hormone therapy was continued (the relationship had ended)

The patient re-presented with a desire for a pregnancy with a new partner. Under anesthesia, the cervical os was identified and the uterine cavity was checked with a 3.5-mm hysteroscope. After the hormones were withdrawn, she had spontaneous menses. Two intrauterine inseminations were undertaken but were difficult. Thereafter, transcervical cannulation was not possible.

IVF was performed using the down-regulation protocol with GnRH agonist and 225 units of recombinant FSH. On day 2, a 2-cell embryo was transferred into the ampulla of the left tube. Pregnancy did not ensue. Subsequently a second IVF with transmyometrial transfer of a day 3 embryo was using the same protocol was again undertaken. Three additional day 3 embryos and a day 5 blastocyst were also cryopreserved. Pregnancy did not ensue with the fresh transfer or with two further transmyometrial transfers using a Towako needle (Cook Ltd., Letchworth, Herts, UK) with its stylet passed through the anterior vaginal fornix, through the myometrium of the anterior uterine wall with its adjacent endometrium, and into the endometrium of the posterior wall. Tubal transfer was undertaken with the last day 3 cryopreserved embryo. Although intrauterine pregnancy occurred, it was nonviable; the patient miscarried at 7 weeks.

The cryopreserved blastocyst was placed in an ovulatory cycle by laparoscopic transfer using a Potter GIFT catheter (Cook Ob/Gyn) introduced 4 to 5 cm into the left tube. An intrauterine pregnancy ensued, and monitoring included regular ultrasound examinations of the cervix and uterus.

At 29 weeks gestation emergency cesarean section was required due to a 3-cm herniation of the uterus posteriorly just above where the tape was observed together with some free fluid in the pelvis.

Outcome

The male infant at birth weighed 1380 g and had a difficult neonatal course with bilateral pneumothoraces. He was discharged after 8 weeks. At age 18 months, he is healthy apart from a minor language delay.

Four months post partum the patient represented with a 5-cm hematometra. High-dose progestogen therapy was administered, with symptomatic relief but no reduction in the hematometra. Two months later, with a recurrence of pelvic cramps, percutaneous drainage of the hematometra was performed using ultrasound-guided needle aspiration under general anesthesia.

A month later, the patient had further pain – the hematometra had recurred. A second aspiration was planned, but overnight the patient developed severe pain requiring hospitalization with an acute abdomen. An ultrasound scan showed reduction of the hematometra and free fluid in the pelvis. At laparotomy, a 1-cm uterine rupture just above the suture was noted, and subtotal hysterectomy with removal of the tape was undertaken. Her recovery was protracted, but after 6 months, she was eventually pain free.

General remarks

This is an example of an alternative route of embryo transfer, namely successful intrafallopian transfer of a blastocyst and of pregnancy after IVF and tubal transfer in a woman who had a laparoscopic cervical cerclage before pregnancy.

The tube in which a cleaved embryo normally develops on days 1 to 3 has a different metabolic environment than the uterus, where on days 4 and 5, the morula and blastocyst develop [1]. Assisted reproductive technologies such as gamete intrafallopian transfer, zygote intrafallopian tube transfer, and tubal transfer of early-stage embryos [2] were introduced in part because the distal tube was presumed to be a better environment than the uterus for the early stages of embryo development [3].

IVF culture media and transcervical transfer techniques have since improved such that tubal transfer techniques are now uncommon. Now the preferred stage of transcervical transfer is as a blastocyst rather than a cleaved embryo, partly because the uterine cavity is considered to provide a better metabolic environment for the blastocyst than does the fallopian tube [2].

Sometimes, however, cannulation of the cervical canal for embryo or blastocyst transfer is not possible. Because tubal transfer usually requires a laparoscopy, transmyometrial transfer under ultrasound guidance is a less invasive option [4].

When cervical transfer is not possible, the usual alternative is transmyometrial replacement. This was attempted twice in this patient, but no pregnancy resulted.

Most of the literature reports on transmyometrial transfers are case reports. There is one published prospective randomized study [5] which compared transmyometrial to traditional transcervical embryo transfer. The pregnancy rate was lower (1/20 vs. 3/20), but the study was clearly underpowered.

A theoretical risk of intrafallopian transfer of a blastocyst is tubal pregnancy, with the blastocyst hatching and implanting before reaching the uterus. The depth of the laparoscopic transfer of 4 to 5 cm was chosen deliberately in the hope that the blastocyst would pass into the uterus within 1 to 2 days. Blastocyst tubal transfer may ultimately prove to have an increased ectopic pregnancy rate, but this case suggests that it is a feasible alternative to transmyometrial transfer when there is cervical obstruction.

The cerclage was associated with imminent uterine rupture during pregnancy, necessitating premature delivery of a very low-birth-weight infant. The subsequent posterior uterine rupture of a hematometra necessitated hysterectomy. Neither of these complications have been reported previously with cervical cerclage.

References

1. Gardner DK, Lane M, Calderon I, Leeton J. Environment of the preimplantation human embryo in vivo: metabolite analysis of oviduct and uterine fluids and metabolism of cumulus cell. *Fertil Steril* 1996; **65**: 349–53.

2. Balmacedan JP, Gastaldi C, Remophi J, Borrero C, Ord T, Asch RH. Tubal embryo transfer as a treatment for infertility due to male factor. *Fertil Steril* 1988; **50**: 476–9.

3. Bulletti C. Debating tubal transfer in assisted reproductive technology. *Hum Reprod* 1996; **11**: 1820–2.

4. Jamal W, Phillips SJ, Hemmings R, Lapensee L, Couturier B, Bissonnette F *et al.* Successful pregnancy following novel IVF protocol and transmyometrial embryo transfer after radical vaginal trachelectomy. *Reprod Biomed Online* 2009; **18**: 700–3.

5. Groutz A, Lessing JB, Wolf Y, Azem F, Yovel I, Amit A. Comparison of transmyometrial and transcervical embryo transfer in patients with previously failed in vitro fertilization–embryo transfer cycles and/or cervical stenosis. *Ferti. Steril* 1997; **67**: 1073–6.

Chapter
27

Mild-approach ART in a patient with polycystic ovary syndrome

Michel De Vos

Clinical fertility history

A 31-year-old woman ("A.") was referred to the fertility clinic because of 6 months of secondary amenorrhea that had arisen after discontinuing the combined oral contraceptive pill (OCP; cyproterone acetate 2 mg + ethinyl estradiol 0.035 mg) to become pregnant. She had never been pregnant before and had been on OCP for almost ten years, during which time she had had monthly withdrawal bleeds. OCP had initially been prescribed to alleviate symptoms of hyperandrogenism.

General medical, family, and social history

Although A. had been properly warned against the increased risk of thromboembolic events in smokers who are taking OCP, she had been a heavy smoker for many years but managed to stop smoking before being referred to the fertility clinic. At the time of presentation she was not taking any drugs but she had been on varenicline to aid her stopping smoking until 6 weeks before attending the fertility clinic. Her surgical history includes a bilateral breast reduction, and because of the history of invasive breast cancer in her mother, who had died at the age of 38, she had undergone mammography at the age of 30, with normal results. Born of Turkish parents, A. was working as an intercultural social worker in a university hospital.

Examination findings

A. had a BMI of 23.0 kg/m² and overt signs of hyperandrogenism, including facial acne vulgaris which she reported to have worsened since cessation of OCP, and excess hair growth resulting in a score of 8 on the Ferriman Gallwey scale. Gynecological examination and Pap smear testing for cervical cytology revealed no abnormalities.

Fertility investigations

A transvaginal ultrasound scan (USS) showed uterine dimensions of 66 × 30 mm, a right ovary measuring 41 × 18 mm and a left ovary measuring 40 × 28 mm. In both ovaries, between 35 and 40 small antral follicles measuring less than 5 mm were observed in the cortex, with dense ovarian stroma (Figure 27.1). The endometrial lining was thin (2 mm). Hormonal profiling showed a normal thyroid function and a circulating prolactin level of 760 mIU/L (with 102–496 mIU/L being the normal range), and confirmed an important degree of hyperandrogenemia, as evidenced by elevated levels of DHEAS (3.57 mg/L [0.99–3.40 mg/L]), androstenedione (4865 ng/L [700–3500 ng/L]), testosterone (0.74 μg/L

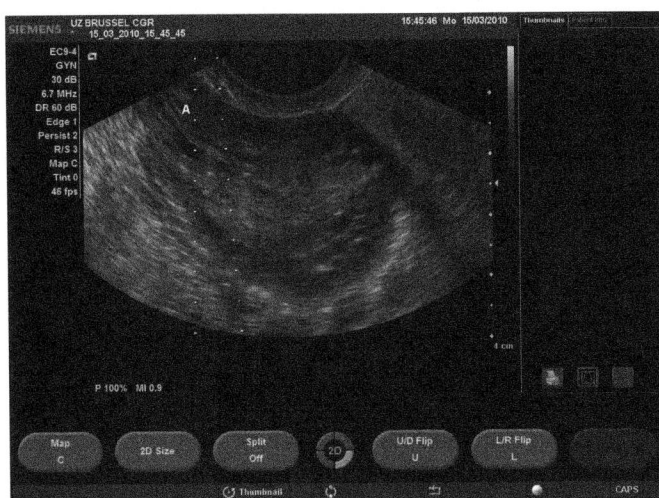

Figure 27.1 Ultrasound findings.

[0.12–0.52 µg/L]), and free testosterone concentration (9.6 ng/L [0.2–6.4 ng/L]). Sperm analysis revealed normal results according to the WHO criteria. Tubal patency testing was not performed.

Diagnosis

Based on amenorrhea, hyperandrogenemia/hyperandrogenism, and polycystic ovarian morphology, A. was diagnosed with polycystic ovary syndrome (PCOS) in accordance with Rotterdam criteria (Rotterdam ESHRE/ASRM-Sponsored PCOS Consensus Workshop Group 2004).

Action plan

In view of the normal sperm count, ovulation induction was attempted using 100 mg of clomiphene citrate for 5 days, after a progestin-induced withdrawal bleeding. On cycle day 11, USS showed no follicular size increase and a blood test yielded the following results: FSH 5.60 IU/L, progesterone 0.92 µg/L, E2 124 ng/L, and LH 24.5 IU/L. Hence, 150 mg of clomiphene was given for a further 5 days. Hormone analysis on the day following cessation of clomiphene showed an FSH serum level of 4.30 IU/L, progesterone 0.74 µg/L, E2 150 ng/L, and LH 17.9 IU/L.

Second-line potential approaches for ovulation induction were discussed with the patient and her partner, including gonadotropins, laparoscopic ovarian drilling, or IVM. The couple consented to undergo IVM treatment, which was preceded by one cycle of OCP. On day 3 of withdrawal bleeding, USS showed an unchanged picture of ovarian morphology and hormone analysis revealed the following results: FSH 0.20 IU/L, progesterone 0.51 µg/L, E2 74 ng/L, and LH 0.20 IU/L. Subsequently, ovarian stimulation was started using 75 IU HP-HMG daily. After 6 days of stimulation, USS showed an endometrium thickness of 4.5 mm and a grossly unchanged antral follicular pattern, with the largest follicles not exceeding 6 mm. Hormonal testing showed the following serum levels: FSH 7.20 IU/L, progesterone 0.65 µg/L, E2 63 ng/L, LH 6.5 IU/L.

Ovarian puncture for egg retrieval was performed on the following day. No hCG trigger was given. Twenty-four cumulus–oocyte complexes were obtained. After 40 hours' IVM, seven oocytes had become mature. After ICSI, four zygotes developed. On day 3 after ICSI, three embryos of good morphology were vitrified electively because of suboptimal endometrial thickness, as described by Guzman *et al.* (2012).

Outcome

After vitrified-warmed transfer of two embryos, A. became pregnant with dizygotic twins. A glucose tolerance test, performed at 24 weeks gestation, showed normal results. The pregnancy was uneventful until 34 weeks and 4 days gestation, when A. was admitted to the labor ward because of premature uterine contractions. Cardiotocography showed signs of fetal distress of one fetus; an emergency cesarean section was performed on the day of admission, resulting in the live birth of a healthy boy, with birth weight 2020 g, and a healthy girl with birth weight 1650 g.

General remarks

Polycystic ovary syndrome is the most common endocrine disorder in women of reproductive age. Rotterdam diagnostic criteria are most widely used to establish the diagnosis, and based on these criteria, the prevalence of PCOS is estimated to be almost 18% (March *et al.* 2010). Hyperandrogenism and anovulatory subfertility are often presenting symptoms, although potential systemic involvement warrants close follow-up during pregnancy and thereafter, in view of the impact of PCOS on glucose metabolism and cardiovascular health. Clomiphene citrate (CC) represents the first-line approach for ovulation induction in patients with PCOS who want to become pregnant (Thessaloniki ESHRE/ASRM-Sponsored PCOS Consensus Workshop Group 2008), and ovulation can be achieved in 75–80% of women with PCOS-related infertility, resulting in a cumulative pregnancy rate of 70–75% after six to nine cycles of treatment (Imani *et al.* 2002). Recent evidence suggests that ovulation induction using gonadotropins results in improved pregnancy rates compared to CC, although this approach often requires more careful monitoring to avoid multiple pregnancy (Homburg *et al.* 2012). Laparoscopic ovarian drilling has also been proposed as a second-line approach in women with PCOS (Gjönnaess 1984). Metformin, an insulin-reducing biguanide, lowers androgen levels and is also capable of restoring ovulation in a subset of anovulatory patients with PCOS. Although conventional ovarian stimulation using gonadotropins, followed by IVF or ICSI, yields excellent pregnancy rates in patients with PCOS (Heijnen *et al.* 2006), this approach may be cumbersome in a subset of patients with very elevated antral follicle count and circulating AMH-levels (Xi *et al.* 2012). Furthermore, patients with PCOS have a particularly increased risk of developing OHSS, although novel methods based on the replacement of hCG as ovulation trigger by a GnRH-agonist can significantly reduce that risk (Radesic and Tremellen 2011). Oocyte in vitro maturation has emerged as a promising ART with great potential in patients with PCOS because it can eliminate OHSS completely and results in fewer side effects than conventional stimulation, because of the minimal use of stimulatory hormones. Nevertheless, pregnancy rates are still low compared with conventional ART (Gremeau *et al.* 2012) and further research is required to improve oocyte competence and endometrial quality in IVM treatment cycles. Pregnant women with PCOS have an increased risk of first trimester pregnancy loss, and of complications such as preeclampsia, premature delivery, and small-for-gestational-age babies.

References

Gjönnaess H. Polycystic ovarian syndrome treated by ovarian electrocautery through the laparoscope. *Fertil Steril* 1984; **41**: 20–5.

Gremeau *et al.* In vitro maturation or in vitro fertilization for women with polycystic ovaries? A case–control study of 194 treatment cycles. *Ferti Steril* 2012; DOI:10.1016/j.fertnstert.2012.04.046.

Guzman *et al.* Developmental capacity of in vitro-matured human oocytes retrieved from polycystic ovary syndrome ovaries containing no follicles larger than 6 mm. *Fertil Steril* 2012; DOI:10.1016/j.fertnstert.2012.01.114.

Heijnen EM, Eijkemans MJ, Hughes EG, Laven JS, Macklon NS, Fauser BC. A meta-analysis of outcomes of conventional IVF in women with polycystic ovary syndrome. *Hum Reprod Update* 2006; **12**: 13–21.

Homburg R, Hendriks ML, Konig TE, Anderson RA, Balen A, Brincat M *et al.* Clomifene citrate of low-dose FSH for the first line treatment of infertile women with anovulation associated with polycystic ovary syndrome: a prospective randomized multinational study. *Hum Reprod* 2012; **27**: 468–73.

Imani B, Eijkemans MJ, te Velde ER, Habbema JD, Fauser BC. A nomogram to predict the probability of live birth after clomiphene citrate induction of ovulation in normogonadotropic oligoamenorrheic infertility. *Fertil Steril* 2002; **77**: 91–7. DOI:10.1016/S0015-0282(01)02929-6.

March WA, Moore VM, Willson KJ, Phillips DI, Norman RJ, Davies MJ. The prevalence of polycystic ovary syndrome in a community sample assessed under contrasting diagnostic criteria. *Hum Reprod* 2010; **25**: 544–51. DOI:10.1093/humrep/dep399.

Radesic B, Tremellen K. Oocyte maturation employing a GnRH agonist in combination with low-dose hCG luteal rescue minimizes the severity of ovarian hyperstimulation syndrome while maintaining excellent pregnancy rates. *Hum Reprod* 2011; **26**(12): 3437–42.

Rotterdam ESHRE/ASRM-Sponsored PCOS Consensus Workshop Group. Revised 2003 consensus on diagnostic criteria and long-term health risks related to polycystic ovary syndrome. *Fertil Steril* 2004; **81**: 19–25.

Thessaloniki ESHRE/ASRM-Sponsored PCOS Consensus Workshop Group. Consensus on infertility treatment related to polycystic ovary syndrome. *Fertil Steril* 2008; **89**: 505–22. DOI:10.1016/j.fertnstert.2007.09.041.

Xi W *et al.* Correlation of serum Anti-Müllerian hormone concentrations on day 3 of the in vitro fertilization stimulation cycle with assisted reproduction outcome in polycystic ovary syndrome patients. *J Assist Reprod Genet* 2012; **29**(5): 397–402. DOI 10.1007/s10815-012-9726-x.

A slim patient with polycystic ovary syndrome (PCOS)

Robert Lahoud, Manveen (Manny) Mangat, and Cherise Mooy

History

Mrs. D.O. first presented to her gynecologist at the age of 30 with a history of 4 months' secondary amenorrhea wanting to conceive. She had her menarche at the age of 14 and her periods were irregular ranging between 28 days and up to 9 months in cycle length. She described her puberty as normal otherwise. At the age of 20 Mrs. D.O. was started on the combined oral contraceptive pill for reasons of contraception and to regulate periods. In her mid-twenties she stopped the oral contraceptive for 6 months. She was diagnosed with polycystic ovary syndrome by an endocrinologist.

At the age of 30 the subject stopped the oral contraceptive again to try to conceive. When she presented with a 4-month history of secondary fertility there was no history of galactorrhea, headaches, or vasomotor symptoms. She complained of mild acne but no hirsutism. There was no history of an eating disorder or other causes of anovulation such as excessive exercise.

On examination Mrs. D.O. had minimal acne and no hirsutism. Her height was 173 cm and her weight was 60 kg, giving her a body mass index (BMI) of 20 kg/m². The physical examination was normal.

Investigations

Ultrasound indicated a normal uterus with an endometrial thickness of 3.4 mm. Both ovaries contained more than 20 peripheral follicles with ovarian volumes greater than 10 mL, classifying them as polycystic.

Blood testing showed the following picture: LH 15.9 IU/L, FSH 6 IU/L, estradiol 279 pmol/L, prolactin 98 mIU/L, thyroid function tests normal, testosterone 1.4 nmol/L, sex hormone-binding globulin 94 nmol/L, and free androgen index 1.5% (normal). The adrenal androgens were normal.

The semen analysis of her partner was normal.

Diagnosis

Polycystic ovary syndrome (PCOS).

The patient has a history menstrual cycle irregularities over several years, polycystic ovaries on ultrasound, and mild acne as well as a raised baseline serum LH concentration. Based on the Rotterdam criteria for diagnosing PCOS, this patient qualifies for this diagnosis. It is important to exclude hypothalamic amenorrhea, which may also present in a similar way in slim patients.

Treatment history

Provera (medroxy progesterone acetate) 10 mg was given for 7 days after a negative pregnancy test. There was no withdrawal bleed following Provera use. Clomiphene citrate at a dose of up to 150 mg for 5 days in the follicular phase did not result in ovulation.

The patient was referred to a reproductive endocrinologist. Clomiphene-resistant PCOS was diagnosed. Ovulation induction treatment using gonadotropins was recommended. About 3 weeks prior to starting FSH the patient was started on metformin 1500 mg/day.

Mrs. D.O. was then started on recombinant follicle-stimulating hormone (rFSH) at a dose of 50 IU/day. A slow step-up protocol was used. After 10 days of FSH the serum estradiol concentration had plateaued at a level of 460 pmol/L and the follicles were not growing on ultrasound (all <10 mm diameter). The rFSH dose was increased to 75 IU per day. Five days later the estradiol level had increased to 1894 pmol/L but the follicles were still small (11 mm leading follicle). Over the next three days, despite the rFSH injections being reduced to 25 IU/day the estradiol level reached 10 760 pmol/L with an ultrasound showing follicles at only 14 mm or less. It was decided to cancel this treatment cycle because of the risk of multiple pregnancy.

A repeat attempt at ovulation induction again was unsuccessful. After 17 days of 50 IU there was no follicular response and on 75 IU an over-response was seen and the attempt was once again abandoned.

After review of the patient and discussion of the risk of multiple pregnancy, it was decided to proceed with in vitro fertilization (IVF). A long down-regulation (LDR) protocol was used to lower LH levels.

After 13 days of 75 IU rFSH per day, an estradiol level of 6966 pmol/L was reached and two leading follicles 18 mm and greater were seen on ultrasound. Recombinant hCG (Ovidrel) 250 µg was given as a trigger injection (36 hours prior to oocyte retrieval).

Twenty oocytes were collected and inseminated with standard IVF techniques. Thirteen embryos formed. On day 5 of culture, one top-quality embryo was transferred (expanded blastocyst AA grade) and three embryos were frozen (slow frozen technique). After standard luteal phase support with progesterone gel, the patient did not conceive and no ovarian hyperstimulation syndrome (OHSS) was experienced.

The following frozen embryo transfer (FET) cycle was started using hormone replacement therapy (HRT) with Progynova (estradiol valerate) 4 mg/day. The embryo survival was poor (expected to be 80%) with only one of the three embryos surviving. Mrs. D.O. again did not conceive.

The second stimulated IVF cycle again involved an LDR protocol. Once again 75 IU of rFSH was used (for 11 days) and this time an estradiol level of 11 000 pmol/L was reached prior to ovulation trigger. Twenty-one oocytes were retrieved, 11 were fertilized, and one top-grade embryo was transferred on day 5 of embryo culture (expanded blastocyst BA). Six top-grade embryos were frozen.

This time, following luteal support using progesterone gel, Mrs. D.O. achieved a positive pregnancy test. The patient developed moderate to severe late-onset OHSS, which was managed on an outpatient basis. The main feature on ultrasound was very enlarged ovaries (11 cm in diameter). There was minor ascites and signs of hemoconcentration with a raised hematocrit level. The level of OHSS could have warranted admission to hospital, except for the patient wanting to manage this at home. As it turned out, the OHSS resolved over the next two weeks and the patient went on to have a straightforward pregnancy. A girl weighing

3560 g was delivered at term by normal vaginal delivery. There were no pregnancy-related complications or fetal anomalies.

The next three FETs were all unsuccessful. Embryo survival was again below average with only 50% of the embryos surviving the freeze–thaw. By now the patient was convinced that frozen embryos were not successful in her case.

Either way, a repeat IVF attempt (third cycle) was performed using an LDR protocol and 75 IU of rFSH. This time an estradiol level of 3400 pmol/L was reached and eight oocytes were collected. three embryos formed and one top-quality blastocyst was transferred. This time there were no embryos to freeze. Despite the more moderate response, the patient developed severe late-onset OHSS requiring one day of hospitalization. She then received "hospital at home" care with intravenous fluids, prophylactic antithrombotic treatment, and antinausea medications. The OHSS resolved after a week and the pregnancy progressed well. A live-born boy weighing 4180 g was born at term by normal vaginal delivery. No fetal anomalies or pregnancy complications were noted.

After two live births, two episodes of OHSS, and four unsuccessful FET cycles, Mrs. D.O. decided to return for baby number three. In 2011 the patient underwent another stimulated IVF cycle. With this cycle cabergoline was added from the time of the transfer to the pregnancy test. Other means to prevent OHSS included metformin (used in previous cycles) and a reduction in rFSH to about 68 IU of FSH. An antagonist cycle was considered, but because of the previous success, the LDR cycle was preferred.

During that cycle the patient did not respond to 8 days of 68 IU of rFSH and after a further 10 days of 75 IU of rFSH an estradiol concentration of 7807 pmol/L was reached. Eighteen oocytes were retrieved and 13 embryos formed. One top-grade blastocyst was transferred and five top-grade blastocysts were frozen. Again Mrs. D.O. conceived but this time she did not develop OHSS. The pregnancy progressed well until the 18-week morphology ultrasound. This showed bilateral renal agenesis and major cardiac anomalies in the fetus. Because of the poor prognosis for the child, a termination of pregnancy was performed. No specific cause for the anomalies was detected and, after genetic counseling, the recurrence risk of such a fetal anomaly was thought to be low.

Mrs. D.O. returned in 2012 for further treatment. The reproductive endocrinologist assured her that it was worth using the frozen embryos. These were vitrified embryos with high survival rates. With the FET protocol for anovulatory patients, the specialist had moved to stimulated FET cycles (higher pregnancy rates). In these cycles a small dose of FSH is used to stimulate the ovaries to induce ovulation. Embryo transfer occurs 5 days after ovulation. The patients are warned of the small risk of multiple pregnancy and in this case advised against having sexual intercourse around the time of ovulation.

A single embryo was transferred 5 days following monofollicular ovulation induced with 62.5 IU of FSH (Gonal F). On ultrasound at 7 weeks a dizygotic pregnancy was recorded. Both twins were delivered at term.

Discussion

Polycystic ovary syndrome is a common endocrine disorder in females of reproductive age. Since the advent of the Rotterdam criteria for the diagnosis of PCOS [1], the prevalence of PCOS has risen. One of the reasons for this is the broader definition including ultrasound findings. Practically this means that a larger number of slim women are now diagnosed with PCOS.

It is important for reproductive endocrinologists to preach the message that obesity does not *have* to be part of the PCOS diagnosis. The case described here highlights that many women with PCOS are slim. The days of diagnosing all cases of PCOS, as the obese patient walks into the consulting rooms, are over.

From a fertility outcome perspective, there have been few studies distinguishing slim PCOS women with overweight ones. Slim PCOS women are more likely to have amenorrhea rather than oligomenorrhea. They have fewer symptoms of hyperandrogenism and biochemical hyperandrogenism is less marked, but most have high baseline LH concentrations. Hence Mrs. D.O. represents the typical phenotype described.

The case outlined in this chapter underscores that when it comes to ovulation induction, slim PCOS patients, understandably, require less gonadotropin to achieve a response. With superovulation for IVF, slim patients are known to be at higher risk of OHSS [2]. Miscarriages are also said to be more common for PCOS patients. Much evidence suggests one of the confounding factors to be obesity, and one wonders whether obstetric risks such as miscarriage are also increased in the slim PCOS patient [3].

The case of Mrs. D.O. shows the typical pathway for treating subfertility in PCOS. Lifestyle modification is the first-line intervention, but is less effective in slim PCOS women. Clomiphene citrate is the first-line pharmacological treatment for ovulation induction. The case of Mrs. D.O. is one of clomiphene resistance. The evaluation of anovulatory women (WHO type 2) revealed that clomiphene resistance was associated with an increased free androgen index (FAI; hyperandrogenemia), elevated body mass index (BMI; obesity), greater mean ovarian volume (as an ultrasound feature of polycystic ovaries), and amenorrhea [4]. Furthermore, studies have suggested that increased serum LH concentration may predict a lesser response to ovulation induction treatment. In this case LH levels were raised, possibly explaining the lack of response to clomiphene citrate.

The case of Mrs. D.O. highlights the difficulties clinicians may face in treating slim women with PCOS. There is a "fine line" between no response and an over response. In this case at a dose of 75 IU of recombinant FSH a large cohort of follicles responded to stimulation. At any smaller dose there was no response. This makes ovulation induction often unsafe, as the risk of multiple pregnancy is too great. With IVF the next risk is that of OHSS.

According to the most recent Cochrane review, laparoscopic ovarian drilling in clomiphene-resistant women has been reported to be associated with a smaller risk of multiple pregnancy compared with the use of gonadotropins. This treatment is certainly a second-line treatment option to be considered. The risk of postoperative complications such as formation of adhesions makes this treatment less attractive.

The case of Mrs. D.O. highlights the link between PCOS and OHSS. The good news is that now there are options in the prevention of OHSS. In this case with the last IVF cycle a combination of metformin, cabergoline, and low-dose FSH stimulation helped to prevent OHSS.

The use of GnRH antagonists in IVF cycles is said to reduce the incidence of OHSS compared with LDR protocols. The greatest advantage of using GnRH antagonist protocols is that a GnRH agonist trigger can be effectively used to essentially eliminate the risk of OHSS to the patient [5]. The decision to use a GnRH agonist can be made late in the ovarian stimulation process when the true risk can be better assessed. Some even advocate the universal use of GnRH agonist trigger and freezing of all embryos. Even though freezing techniques for embryos have greatly improved in the last decade, the current case highlights one of the problems clinicians may face with low survival of frozen embryos. In conclusion, a flexible approach offered in a GnRH antagonist cycle utilizing the OHSS prevention methods mentioned above would constitute the modern IVF management for PCOS women.

Hence, one measure to prevent OHSS must be to diagnose PCOS prior to starting a cycle with high-quality ultrasound and antimüllerian hormone testing. A patient deemed at risk of OHSS should be stimulated with a low-dose FSH regime and a GnRH antagonist protocol.

In summary, the case of Mrs. D.O. highlights the difficulties of ovulation induction and the fact that OHSS is not always preventable. It can be managed successfully and safely. Finally, most women with PCOS will succeed with treatment and will go on to have a family.

References

1. Rotterdam ESHRE/ASRM-Sponsored PCOS consensus workshop group. Revised 2003 consensus on diagnostic criteria and long-term health risks related to polycystic ovary syndrome (PCOS). *Human Reproduction* 2004; **19**(1): 41–7.

2. Nastri CO, Ferriani RA, Rocha IA, Martins WP. Ovarian hyperstimulation syndrome: pathophysiology and prevention. *Journal of Assisted Reproduction and Genetics* 2010; **27**(2–3): 121–8.

3. Wang JX, Davies MJ, Norman RJ. Polycystic ovarian syndrome and the risk of spontaneous abortion following assisted reproductive technology treatment. *Human Reproduction* 2001; **16**(12): 2606–9.

4. Eijkemans MJ, Habbema JD, Fauser BC. Characteristics of the best prognostic evidence: an example on prediction of outcome after clomiphene citrate induction of ovulation in normogonadotropic oligoamenorrheic infertility. *Semin Reprod Med* 2003; **21**(1): 39–47.

5. Humaidan P, Papanikolaou EG, Kyrou D, Alsbjerg B, Polyzos NP, Devroey P, Fatemi HM. The luteal phase after GnRH-agonist triggering of ovulation: present and future perspectives. *Reproductive Biomedicine Online* 2012; **24**(2): 134–41.

Chapter

29

Recurrent cycles with retrieval of immature germinal vesicle (GV) oocytes

Sonal Karia, Mark Bowman, and Derek Lok

Introduction

The aim of controlled ovarian stimulation in IVF cycles is to ensure the collection of fully mature oocytes that are at the metaphase II stage. However, in some cases immature or maturing oocytes are recovered from follicles and often do not complete maturation in vitro. When such outcomes occur recurrently, it poses a unique challenge and a case demonstrating this is discussed here.

History and examination

A 31-year-old para 1 woman presented to the fertility clinic at Royal Prince Alfred Hospital in NSW, Australia in February 2009 with a history of secondary infertility for 2 years. She had had a natural conception about 6 years prior to presentation, resulting in the birth of a healthy male child weighing 4.07 kg via lower-segment cesarean section for failure to progress in labor. The pregnancy was complicated by insulin-requiring gestational diabetes mellitus. She was using combined OCP for contraception for the first three years after the birth of her first child. She had 28- to 35- day menstrual cycles lasting for 5 to 7 days with moderate dysmenorrhea for the previous year without history of dyspareunia, dysuria, or dyschezia. There was no history of intermenstrual or postcoital bleeding. She was aware of her fertile period and had regular intercourse (2–3 times per week) with her partner. There was no other significant past medical, surgical, social, or family history of note for her or her partner. She had attempted three cycles of ovulation induction with clomiphene prior to presentation but no information was available about the ovulation outcome in these cycles.

On examination, she had a high BMI of 39.6 kg/m². There were no other significant findings on systemic or pelvic examination. Examination findings for her partner were unremarkable.

Investigations

Her pelvic ultrasound scan revealed polycystic ovaries with a normal-sized uterus and an endometrial polyp measuring 4.6 mm, with bilateral patent fallopian tubes on Hycosy.

Her hormonal investigations were as follows. Day 1 of cycle:

- FSH 3.0 U/L
- LH 1.6 U/L
- Estradiol <100 pmol/L
- Testosterone 1.0 nmol/L
- SHBG 21.1 nmol/L

- Free androgen index 4.7
- 17-Hydroxyprogesterone 3.7 nmol/L
- Antenatal screen – nil abnormality detected

Her partner's semen analysis results were as follows:

- Volume 7 mL
- Sperm concentration 50.8 million/mL
- Motility 55% (rapid 24%, slow 18%, nonprogressive 13%)
- Morphology 15% normal forms
- Trial wash 16 million yield with 72% progressive motility

The partner's serology showed nil abnormality detected.

Management

After detailed discussion of fertility treatment options, a plan was made to proceed with IVF. Prior to IVF, the patent underwent a hysteroscopy with polypectomy and uterine curettage revealing secretory endometrium with benign endometrial polyps on histopathology in March 2009.

Her first IVF cycle was carried out in December 2009 using long down-regulation protocol (LDR) with Provera + Synarel + 200 units of FSH + Ovidrel 250 μg for trigger. Eight oocytes were retrieved of which seven were immature with failed fertilization.

In February 2010, a hystero-laparoscopy was performed revealing multiple endometrial polyps leading to polypectomy. The uterus, tubes, ovaries, and pelvis were normal on laparoscopy. In December 2010, the patient underwent laparoscopic band surgery in an attempt to lose weight. Her BMI came down to 34 kg/m² in the month as surgery and a decision to continue ART after another 4–6 months was made. She underwent two more cycles of IVF as follows:

- October 2011 – ICSI
  - LDR with Provera + Synarel + 250 units FSH + trigger with Ovidrel 250 μg
  - 8 oocytes retrieved, all GV, not inseminated
- January 2012 – ICSI
  - 250 units of FSH + Ganirelix 250 μg from day 5
  - Pregnyl 5000 units for trigger
  - 7 oocytes retrieved, all GV, not inseminated

The above outcomes were discussed extensively at the departmental clinical meeting in view of the unexpected outcomes on a background of past spontaneous conception, and a decision was made to proceed with ICSI using antagonist cycle + 250 units FSH + GnRH agonist trigger hoping to achieve natural LH surge instead of using hCG as LH surrogate.

The cycle was carried out in March 2012 as decided, resulting in retrieval of four oocytes (one MII and rest immature). One 4-cell grade 1 embryo was transferred on day 2. The luteal phase was supported with 1500 units of hCG on days 2 and 6, together with 90 mg of progesterone gel vaginally daily. Her hCG level on day 14 after embryo transfer was 283 IU. A viability scan at 6 weeks revealed a single intrauterine gestation corresponding to 5 weeks and 6 days with a FHR of 130 bpm. Unfortunately, the pregnancy ended in a spontaneous complete miscarriage between 13 and 14 weeks gestation.

Two more cycles were attempted with the same protocol; one cycle was cancelled due to premature ovulation prior to pick-up. In the second cycle, one oocyte was retrieved followed by transfer of an 8-cell grade 1 embryo on day 3 but did not result in a pregnancy.

Discussion

Failure to reinitiate meiosis in vivo may occur due to absent or incomplete LH effect, deranged signaling mechanisms, or intrinsic oocyte factors. Numerous researchers have reported similar cases in the literature. Although our patient responded to a change in stimulation protocol in one cycle, there is no consensus on a therapeutic approach that could be suggested for these patients. The utilization of an endogenous LH surge using either a natural cycle IVF or a stimulatory cycle that allows for a natural surge seems to be a logical approach in patients not responding to an LH surrogate, i.e., hCG. This was particularly applicable to our patient knowing that she had had a spontaneous conception resulting in a live birth in the past, suggestive of adequate in vivo maturation of her oocytes. Although distinctly different from the issue being discussed here, a similar approach has been used in patients with recurrent cycles and empty follicle syndrome with limited success. There is a suggestion that some patients may need a longer exposure to trigger for COCs to detach from the follicular wall, and there have been reports of successful recovery of oocytes 24 hours after an initial unsuccessful oocyte collection in the presence of a normal serum hCG and progesterone. Approaches like in vitro maturation, extended culture, ICSI of donor cytoplasm, or maturation-promoting factors are currently being researched and await validation for clinical application in this particular subset of patients.

Further reading

Chen ZQ, Ming TX, Nielsen HI. Maturation arrest of human oocytes at GV stage. *J Hum Reprod Sci* 2012; **3**(3): 153–7.

Hourvitz A, Maman E, Brengauz M, Machtinger R, dor J. Invitro maturation for patients with repeated invitro fertilization failure due to "oocyte maturation abnormalities." *Fertil Steril* 2010; **94**: 496–501.

Lee JE, Kim SD, Jee BC, Suh CS, Kim SH. Oocyte maturity in repeated ovarin stimulation. *Clin Exp Reprod Med* 2011; **38**(4): 234–7.

Levran D, Farhi J, Nahum H, Glezerman M, Weissman A. Maturation arrest of human oocytes as a cause of infertility. *Hum Reprod* 2002; **17** (6): 1604–9.

Lok F, Pritchard J, Lashen H. Successful treatment of empty follicle syndrome by triggering endogenous LH surge using GnRH agonist in an antagonist down-regulated IVF cycle. *Hum Reprod* 2003; **18** (10): 2079–81.

Mrazek M, Fulka J Jr. Failure of oocyte maturation: Possible mechanisms for oocyte maturation arrest. *Hum Reprod* 2003; **18** (11): 2249–52.

Think heterotopic pregnancy

Amanda Kallen and Pasquale Patrizio

Clinical fertility history

M.G. was a 33-year-old gravida 2 para 1 with secondary infertility of one year's duration. After unremarkable fertility testing, including a normal semen analysis and confirmation of patent fallopian tubes by hysterosalpingography, she underwent ovulation induction with clomiphene citrate, hCG trigger, and timed intercourse. Eighteen days after hCG trigger, the hCG level was 943 IU, rising to 2038 IU after 48 hours. She was scheduled for a transvaginal ultrasound, but at 5+0 weeks gestational age presented with painless vaginal spotting.

General medical, family, and social history

M.G. was healthy with a BMI of 24.2 kg/m² and no medical problems or surgical history. She had reported an uncomplicated, spontaneous vaginal delivery 3 years previously and reported no difficulty conceiving at that time. She denied sexually transmitted infections and reports normal, up-to-date Pap smears. She and her husband were both employed in law enforcement. Her family history was notable for hypertension in her father and type I diabetes in her sister; both parents were alive and well and she had no other siblings.

Examination findings

On examination, M.G. had normal vital signs and appeared comfortable. The abdomen was soft and nontender. Bimanual examination revealed a 6-week-size retroverted uterus with no palpable adnexal masses; scant dark blood was present in the vaginal vault.

A transvaginal ultrasound was performed, which revealed a retroverted uterus measuring 10.0 × 6.3 × 7.8 cm and a single gestational sac measuring 1.2 × 1.0 × 1.6 cm with a yolk sac present (see Figure 30.1). An adjacent subchorionic hemorrhage was seen, abutting less than 25% of the gestational sac diameter. Also seen were several well-circumscribed hypoechoic myomas, the largest a posterior lower uterine segment submucosal myoma measuring 1.3 × 1.4 cm. Both adnexa were markedly enlarged, with anechoic cysts measuring up to 6 cm. The left ovary measured 8.9 × 8.5 × 5.9 cm with a corpus luteal cyst and normal arterial flow. The right ovary measured 8.4 × 7.5 × 5.6 cm with a hemorrhagic corpus luteal cyst. Notably, there was an ectopic pregnancy adjacent to the right ovary with a gestational sac measuring 0.6 × 0.7 × 0.7 cm and a yolk sac present. No free fluid was seen. hCG was 10 800 IU.

Her hematocrit was 36.8 mg/dL; the remainder of M.G.'s laboratory results were normal.

Other clinical investigations

After reviewing the available options and confirming with the patient that the pregnancy was desired, the decision was made to proceed with a diagnostic laparoscopy on the basis

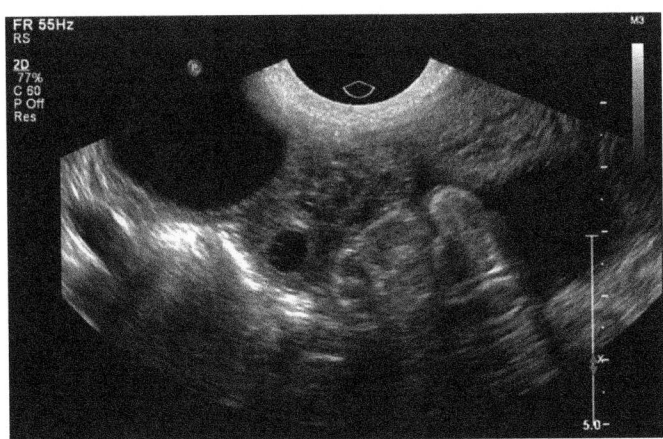

Figure 30.1 Transvaginal ultrasound revealing an ectopic gestational sac adjacent to a viable intrauterine pregnancy.

of suspicion of heterotopic pregnancy. A bulge in the right fallopian tube was noted and a salpingostomy was performed with complete removal of trophoblastic tissue. The patient was discharged the same day. Pathology confirmed chorionic villi and implantation site trophoblasts.

Diagnosis

Heterotopic pregnancy after ovulation induction with clomiphene citrate.

Action plan

Diagnostic laparoscopy and right salpingostomy, with weekly serial ultrasounds to confirm viability of the intrauterine pregnancy.

Outcome

On postoperative day 7, at 6 weeks gestational age, the patient was seen for a postoperative visit. Incisions were healing well. Repeat transvaginal ultrasonography revealed a crown–rump length of 7.1 mm, consistent with gestational age. A fetal heartbeat was present at 140 bpm. Bilateral ovarian cysts were again noted, diminished in size, and no adnexal mass was seen.

General remarks

Heterotopic pregnancy is defined as the simultaneous occurrence of intrauterine and ectopic pregnancies (Luo *et al.* 2009). The incidence of heterotopic pregnancy after spontaneous conception has been reported at around 1 in 30 000; the incidence rises considerably after IVF-ET to up to 1 in 100 (Tal *et al.* 1996). Diagnosis of heterotopic pregnancy may be difficult due to the presence of a concurrent intrauterine gestation. Patients can present with abdominal pain or vaginal bleeding, but in many cases heterotopic pregnancy is asymptomatic and a high index of suspicion is essential. Treatment should be prompt to avoid maternal morbidity and mortality.

Risk factors for heterotopic pregnancy are similar to those for ectopic pregnancy: a history of tubal disease or tubal surgery or prior ectopic pregnancy. However, heterotopic pregnancy can occur in the absence of risk factors (Barrenetxea *et al.* 2007). The incidence following IVF-ET is directly related to the number of embryos transferred (Luo *et al.* 2009). Other factors that may contribute to ectopic include excess media or excess pressure used during transfer, rapid ejection of embryos from the catheter, and misplacement of the transfer catheter (Luo *et al.* 2009). In all ART pregnancies, early ultrasound (at 4–6 weeks gestational age) with systematic examination of the adnexa is recommended, as hCG levels are often unhelpful (they may be elevated due to the presence of two gestations, but may be normal as well).

In the majority of cases associated with ART, the patient will wish to continue the intrauterine pregnancy. In such cases, selective reduction of the ectopic pregnancy may be accomplished via laparoscopy (preferable) or laparotomy. The safety of laparoscopy in pregnancy is well documented (Barrenetxea *et al.* 2007). If the ectopic pregnancy is accessible for injection, methotrexate and/or potassium chloride injection into the gestational sac is an option. Surgical evacuation of the cervical ectopic pregnancy has been reported, and in one case a cerclage was used for control of bleeding. Expectant management is strongly discouraged. In cases where the intrauterine pregnancy is not desired, medical therapy with methotrexate is an option. Methotrexate may be dosed systemically or locally and should be accompanied by curettage to treat the intrauterine gestation. Termination of both pregnancies by administration of methotrexate into the uterine artery and subsequent embolization has also been reported (Faschingbauer *et al.* 2011).

Outcomes after treatment of heterotopic pregnancy are generally, but not always, favorable. In a case series of 12 patients with heterotopic pregnancy after IVF-ET, continuation of pregnancy was observed in 66.7% of patients treated with laparotomy and in both patients treated with selective reduction under ultrasound guidance (Luo *et al.* 2009). However, in a review of CDC data on 132 867 ART pregnancies (of which 207 were heterotopic), heterotopic pregnancies were 30% less likely to result in a live-birth delivery than intrauterine-only pregnancies (Clayton *et al.* 2007).

References

Barrenetxea G, Barinaga-Rementeria L, Lopez de Larruzea A, Agirregoikoa JA, Mandiola M, Carbonero K. Heterotopic pregnancy: Two cases and a comparative review. *Fertility and Sterility* 2007; 87(2): 417.e9–15. DOI: 10.1016/j.fertnstert.2006.05.085.

Clayton HB, Schieve LA, Peterson HB, Jamieson DJ, Reynolds MA, Wright VC. A comparison of heterotopic and intrauterine-only pregnancy outcomes after assisted reproductive technologies in the united states from 1999 to 2002. *Fertility and Sterility* 2007; 87(2): 303–9. DOI: 10.1016/j.fertnstert.2006.06.037.

Faschingbauer F, Mueller A, Voigt F, Beckmann MW, Goecke TW. Treatment of heterotopic cervical pregnancies. *Fertility and Sterility* 2011; 95(5): 1787.e9–13. DOI: 10.1016/j.fertnstert.2010.10.043.

Luo X, Lim CE, Huang C, Wu J, Wong WS, Cheng NC. Heterotopic pregnancy following in vitro fertilization and embryo transfer: 12 cases report. *Archives of Gynecology and Obstetrics* 2009; 280(2): 325–9. DOI: 10.1007/s00404-008-0910-2.

Tal J, Haddad S, Gordon N, Timor-Tritsch I. Heterotopic pregnancy after ovulation induction and assisted reproductive technologies: a literature review from 1971 to 1993. *Fertility and Sterility* 1996; 66(1): 1–12.

Chapter

31

A woman with a hydrosalpinx

Biljana Popovic Todorovic and Gordana Ivanovic

Clinical fertility history

A 32-year-old patient, with a regular menstrual cycle of 26–28 days, presented to a tertiary referral center with a 5-year history of primary infertility due to a previously diagnosed tubal factor. Hysterosalpingography had revealed bilateral tubal blockage, with evident right hydrosalpinx. Laparoscopy was performed with adhesiolysis and liberation of both ovaries; two benign ovarian cysts were removed, and partial omentectomy and myomectomy were carried out as well as partial resection of the right tube.

The patient progressed to have four IVF treatments over a period of two years. All employed flexible GnRH antagonist protocols and different gonadotropin stimulation regimens but a consistent starting dose of 225 IU/day. Eleven to fifteen oocytes were retrieved; on average seven embryos developed after ICSI, and no pregnancy occurred. In the first attempt IVF vs. ICSI was done and no fertilization occurred following IVF; consequently only ICSI was performed.

General medical, family, and social history and examination findings

The patient had a body mass index of 21 kg/m². A pelvic examination revealed normal external genitalia and bimanual examination revealed no pelvic tenderness and a uterus enlarged by the presence of a fibroid on the posterior wall.

She reported that in the second half of the menstrual cycle she often had fluidly discharge which occasionally intensified as menstrual cycle bleeding approached.

Fertility investigations

An ultrasound on day 3 of the cycle was performed which revealed an antral follicle count of 6 on the right ovary and 5 on the left ovary. The uterus was enlarged by the presence of posterior wall fibroid 45 × 38 mm in diameter. She was scanned on a number of occasions during the menstrual cycle, and a scan on day 14 revealed postovulatory finding and an evident right hydrosalpinx.

Basal hormonal status was as follows: FSH 8.7 mIU/mL, LH 5.89 mU/mL, estradiol 36.2 pg/mL, progesterone 0.274 ng/mL, prolactin 191 mIU/L, AMH 1.340 ng/mL, TSH 1.84 μIU/mL. The husband's sperm was reported to have a concentration of 44 million/mL, with total motility of 40%.

Action plan

The patient was advised to undergo surgical removal of hydrosalpinx and myomectomy. Laparotomy was performed, due to the previous surgery, with right salpingectomy and myomectomy.

Outcome

Following recovery, the patient progressed to her fifth IVF attempt. Ovarian stimulation was performed in a long GnRH agonist protocol, with hMG at a starting dose of 300 IU. The dose remained unchanged during the course of stimulation. Eleven COCs were retrieved with 11 MII oocytes; eight were fertilized with ICSI and on day 3 three embryos were transferred and two blastocysts were frozen on day 5. Natural micronized progesterone was used for luteal phase support at a dose of 600 mg/daily. An uneventful twin pregnancy followed.

General remarks

Hydrosalpinges are found in 10–30% of all patients undergoing IVF [1]. Tubal disease, especially hydrosalpinges, shows poorer IVF-ET results compared with tubal factor patients without hydrosalpinges [2, 3]. The probability of achieving pregnancy in the presence of hydrosalpinx is decreased by half and even if the pregnancy is achieved the incidence of spontaneous abortion is increased [2, 3]. In particular, hydrosalpinges visible on ultrasound have a detrimental effect on IVF. Patients associated with the poorest prognosis during IVF treatment [4, 5]. The presence of hydrosalpinges affects the outcome of IVF-ET by having an impact on endometrial environment, possibly through the tubo-uterine reflux of hydrosalpinx fluid, which disrupts implantation [6].

The latest Cochrane review concludes that surgical treatment should be considered for all patients with hydrosalpinges prior to IVF treatment [7]. Laparoscopic tubal occlusion is an alternative to laparoscopic salpingectomy in improving pregnancy rates following IVF. More studies need to be conducted in order to assess the value of aspiration of hydrosalpinges prior to IVF [7].

In patients where laparoscopy is contraindicated due to extensive pelvic adhesions, the placement of tubal blocking inserts has recently been investigated [8, 9]. Although the number of patients is relatively small, the results of preliminary studies would suggest that this approach may be an option in patients at increased risk of surgical complications.

Although the primary aim of the surgical procedure in this patient was to treat the hydrosalpinx, myomectomy was also performed. The fibroid, which was < 5 cm, did not distort the uterine cavity. In a prospective study by Khalaf et al., it was shown that small intramural fibroids are associated with a significant reduction in the cumulative pregnancy, ongoing pregnancy, and live birth rates in women undergoing three cycles of IVF/ICSI compared with controls [10].

In conclusion, this case report shows a detrimental effect of hydrosalpinx on the outcome of IVF treatment. All patients should be counseled for surgical treatment of hydrosalpinges before embarking upon IVF treatment.

References

1. Andersen AN, Lindhard A, Loft A et al. The infertile patient with hydrosalpinges. IVF with or without salpingectomy? *Hum Reprod* 1996; **11**: 2081–4.

2. Zeyneloglu HB, Arici A, Olive DL. Adverse effects of hydrosalpinx on pregnancy rates after in vitro fertilization–embryo transfer. *Fertil Steril* 1998; **70**: 492–9.

3. Camus E, Poncelet C, Goffinet F et al. Pregnancy rates after IVF in cases of tubal infertility with and without hydrosalpinx: meta-analysis of published comparative studies. *Hum Reprod* 1999; **14**: 1243–9.

4. De Wit W, Gowrising CJ, Kuik DJ, Lens JW, Schats R. Only hydrosalpinges visible on ultrasound are associated with reduced implantation and pregnancy rates after in vitro fertilization. *Hum Reprod* 1998; **13**: 1696–701.

5. Strandell A, Lindhard A, Waldenstrom U, Thorburn J. Hydrosalpinx and IVF outcome: cumulative results after salpingectomy in a randomized controlled trial. *Hum Reprod* 2001; **16**: 2403–10.

6. Strandell A. The influence of hydrosalpinx on IVF and embryo transfer: a review. *Hum Reprod Update* 2000; **6**: 387–95.

7. Johnson NP, van Voorst S, Sowter MC, Strandell A, Mol BW. Surgical treatment for tubal disease in women due to undergo in vitro fertilization. *Cochrane Database Syst Rev* 2010; (1): CD002125.

8. Galen DI, Khan N, Richter KS. Essure multicenter off label treatment from hydrosalpinx before in vitro fertilization. *J Minim Invasive Gynecol* 2011; **18**(3): 332–42.

9. Mijatovic V, Dreyer K, Emanuel MH et al. Essure hydrosalpinx occlusion prior to IVF-ET as an alternative to laparoscopic salpingectomy. *Eur J Obstet Gynecol Reprod Biol* 2012; **161**(1): 42–5.

10. Khalaf Y, Ross C, El-Toukhy T et al. The effect of small intramural uterine fibroids on the cumulative outcome of assisted conception. *Hum Reprod* 2006; **21**(10): 2640–4.

A PCOS patient with microprolactinoma, autoimmune thyroid disease, and congenital thrombophilia

Biljana Popovic Todorovic and Jelena Todorovic

Clinical fertility history

A 37-year-old patient with a regular menstrual cycle of 28–30 days was seen at a tertiary referral center with a 3-year history of secondary infertility. Four years previously laparoscopy had been performed, revealing a normal uterus and ovaries and patent fallopian tubes. The following year she conceived a spontaneous pregnancy which ended in a missed abortion at 6 weeks gestation.

Due to a progressively worsening sperm count, a year later an IVF/ICSI treatment was performed in another center, using a long GnRH agonist protocol with a starting dose of 225 IU of recFSH. Fourteen oocytes were retrieved and three day 2 embryos were transferred. Early OHSS developed and the patient was hospitalized 4 days following embryo transfer, for 9 days. hCG testing was positive, but the patient started bleeding and although ectopic pregnancy was suspected, hCG dropped levels spontaneously.

Having failed to conceive again another year later, the patient underwent repeat laparoscopy and hysteroscopy was also performed. Once again, normally sized and positioned uterus and ovaries were observed, and both tubes were of normal morphology, free of adhesions, and patent. Hysteroscopy revealed a discrete fundal impression and in the region of left tubal opening, an endometrial polyp which was removed. She then presented to our clinic.

General medical, family, and social history and examination findings

The patient had a family history of diabetes mellitus type 2. Her body mass index was 24.1 kg/m². A pelvic examination revealed normal external genitalia and bimanual examination revealed no pelvic tenderness and masses.

She reported having gone through menarche at the age of 13 years. At the age of 22, her periods became irregular, with intervals of up to 80 days. Elevated prolactin levels led to the MRI diagnosis of microprolactinoma. Bromocriptine at a maximum dose of 7.5 mg/day was prescribed, and at her last MRI follow-up at 32 years of age, the tumor had regressed and she had been on a maintenance dose of 1.25 mg since then.

Following her first IVF/ICSI attempt, the patient had been reviewed by an endocrinologist, and a glucose tolerance test led to metformin therapy and dietary changes which led to a 15 kg body weight reduction.

There was also a history of autoimmune thyroid disease as a result of thyreoiditis chronica lymphocitaria. Thyroid peroxidase (TPO) and thyroglobulin (TG) antibodies were elevated but the TSH level was within the normal range for pregnancy.

Fertility investigations

An ultrasound scan on day 3 of the cycle was performed which showed an antral follicle count of 13 on the right ovary and 14 on the left ovary. Both ovaries demonstrated polycystic features. Basal hormonal status was as follows: FSH 5.6 mIU/mL, LH 5.8 mU/mL, estradiol 28.3 pg/mL, progesterone 0.565 ng/mL, prolactin 211 mIU/L, AMH 3.65 ng/mL, TSH 2.28 μIU/mL. TPO antibodies were 159.8 IU/mL and TG antibodies were 466.6 mIU/mL.

The husband's sperm was found to have a concentration of just 0.6 million/mL of which 38% was motile.

Other clinical investigations

Thrombophilia testing was carried out for protein C, protein S, activated protein C resistance, lupus anticoagulant, anticardiolipin antibodies IgM and IgG, PCR for FII 20210, factor V Leiden, and C677T for MTHFR. A heterozygotic mutation in the gene for factor V Leiden was found. There were no mutations in the genes for MTHFR, C766T, and factor II (prothrombin II, G20210A). All other results were within the normal range.

Diagnosis and action plan

Prior to undergoing further IVF treatment in our center, the patient was assessed by a hematologist and low-molecular-weight heparin (LMWH) therapy was planned. Moreover, due to the previous early pregnancy loss in the presence of auto-immune thyroid disease, levothyroxine in low doses and supplementation of selenium were commenced.

Outcome

The patient then proceeded to IVF using a long agonist protocol, but given her previous history of OHSS, a lower fixed dose of 112.5 IU recFSH was administered. Fifteen cumulus–oocyte complexes (COCs) were retrieved with 14 MII oocytes. Thirteen were fertilized with ICSI; two embryos were transferred and four blastocysts were frozen. Luteal phase support of natural micronized progesterone 200 mg was taken vaginally three times daily. On the day of oocyte retrieval LMWH had been commenced at a dose of 2500 IU/24 h. This dose was increased to 5000 IU/24 h following embryo transfer. The patient conceived, and at 7 weeks a singleton viable pregnancy was confirmed on ultrasound. The patient was closely monitored by the hematologist throughout the whole pregnancy. She developed gestational diabetes, and cesarean section was performed at week 38 resulting in the birth of a healthy baby boy.

General remarks

The continuing trend to delay childbirth means that concurrent conditions are more frequently present, complicating the management of IVF. This 37-year-old patient presented with a history of microprolactinoma, PCOS, and autoimmune thyroid disease and was also found to have a common congenital thrombophilia.

Her hyperprolactinemia was well controlled at presentation on 1.25 mg daily of bromo-criptine, and she was also taking metformin. The use of insulin-sensitizing agents in women with polycystic ovary syndrome who are undergoing IVF treatment cycles has been widely studied. The most recent Cochrane review [1] indicated that the use of metformin lowers the risk of OHSS. The patient had developed early OHSS in her first IVF treatment cycle after being treated with a long protocol and a relatively high dose of FSH. Although GnRH antagonist protocols reduce the risk of OHSS in PCOS [2], this patient was protected by administering a low dose of recFSH in a long agonist protocol. A pregnancy was achieved and no OHSS ensued.

Autoimmune thyroid disease (AITD) *per se* (i.e., without evident thyroid dysfunction) does not appear to compromise pregnancy success rates, but women with AITD are reported to be at an increased risk of miscarriage after ART. Controlled ovarian stimulation leads to an additional strain on the thyroid, especially in women with AITD. Although thyroid function changes after controlled ovarian stimulation are unable to predict the pregnancy outcome, thyroid function should be monitored closely and corrected when necessary.

A number of studies have shown a high prevalence of AITD in polycystic ovary syndrome [3], justifying systematic screening for thyroid disorders in PCOS [4].

Levothyroxine seems to lower the risk for miscarriage and preterm birth in women with thyroid autoimmunity but this is based on only three small studies [5]. Given its high prevalence, there is a need for randomized controlled trials to study the effects of treatment with levothyroxine on pregnancy outcomes. Supplementation of selenium also shows promising results in the AITD population [6].

A further question arising from this case is whether screening for hereditary thrombophilia is indicated after one early pregnancy loss. Kasparova *et al.* examined thrombophilic mutations in a sample of 100 women with at least one miscarriage, showing that the frequency of thrombophilic mutations in the group of women with early pregnancy loss is 1.5–3 times higher than in the general population. Heterozygous mutations of factor V occurred 1.8 times more frequently in the early pregnancy loss group [7].

Our patient was revealed to be heterozygous for factor V Leiden mutation and was treated with LMWH [8] by a hematologist who was closely involved prior to and following IVF treatment, throughout the pregnancy and delivery. This case highlights the benefits of a multidisciplinary approach to the medically complicated IVF patient.

References

1. Tso LO, Costello MF, Albuquerque LE *et al.* Metformin treatment before and during IVF or ICSI in women with polycystic ovary syndrome. *Cochrane Database Syst Rev* 2009;(2): CD006105. DOI: 10.1002/14651858.CD006105.pub2.

2. Mancini F, Tur R, Martinez F *et al.* Gonadotrophin-releasing hormone-antagonists vs long agonist in in-vitro fertilization patients with polycystic ovary syndrome: a meta-analysis. *Gynecol Endocrinol* 2011; 27(3): 150–5.

3. Kachuei M, Jafari F, Kachuei A, Keshteli AH. Prevalence of autoimmune thyroiditis in patients with polycystic ovary syndrome. *Arch Gynecol Obstet* 2012; 285(3): 853–6.

4. Janssen OE, Mehlmauer N, Hahn S *et al.* High prevalence of autoimmune thyroiditis in patients with polycystic ovary syndrome. *Eur J Endocrinol* 2004; 150(3): 363–9.

5. Vissenberg R, van den Boogaard E, van Wely M *et al.* Treatment of thyroid disorders before conception and in early

pregnancy: a systematic review. *Hum Reprod Update* 2012; **18**(4): 360–73.

6. Drutel A, Archambeaud F, Caron P. Selenium and the thyroid gland: more good news for clinicians. *Clin Endocrinol (Oxf)* 2013; **78**(2): 155–64. DOI: 10.1111/cen.12066.

7. Kasparova D, Vrablik M, Fait T. Is screening for hereditary thrombophilia indicated in first early pregnancy loss? *Neuro Endocrinol Lett* 2012; **33**: 76–80.

8. Glueck CJ, Gogenini S, Munjal J et al. Factor V Leiden mutation: a treatable etiology for sporadic and recurrent pregnancy loss. *Fertil Steril* 2008; **89**: 410–16.

IVF outcome in the same patient before and after myomectomy

Hammed A. Tijani and Ying Cheong

Clinical fertility history

A 39-year-old manager presented with a 2-year history of secondary subfertility. She had previously had an uncomplicated termination of pregnancy at the age of 24. Her menstrual history reported heavy but regular periods with occasional mid-cycle bleeding. Her cervical smear tests had been normal.

General medical, family, and social history

The patient had suffered a pulmonary embolism while on the combined oral contraceptive pill 15 years prior to presentation, for which she had received warfarin treatment for 6 months. A thrombophilia screen performed at that time revealed no abnormality. She reported drinking 10 units of alcohol per week but denied smoking. Her husband was fit and well and presented with no significant medical history.

Examination findings

There were no remarkable findings on physical examination.

Fertility investigations

The hormone profile was normal with ovulatory mid-luteal phase progesterone 32 nmol/L. Her antimüllerian hormone level was 7 pmol/L. Pelvic ultrasound scan showed a retroverted uterus measuring 84 × 71 × 85 mm, with an intramural fundal fibroid of size 74 × 49 × 58 mm abutting the uterine cavity. The endometrium was difficult to visualize clearly due to the fibroid but appeared smooth and regular with a thickness of 6 mm. Both ovaries appeared normal.

The husband's semen analysis was normal with concentration of 110 million/mL, 6% normal form, and motility of 64%.

Other clinical investigations

A diagnostic hysteroscopy performed showed an enlarged uterine cavity. The fibroid appeared to be completely intramural, and did not distort the endometrial lining. Laparoscopy showed an enlarged uterus but the pelvis was essentially normal, the fallopian tubes were bilaterally patent, and both ovaries were normal.

Diagnosis

Subfertility associated with uterine fibroids and history of pulmonary embolism while taking oral contraception.

Action plan

The clinical points discussed surrounded a number of issues: (1) the potential impact of a fibroid uterus on subfertility and assisted conception; (2) the need for thromboprophylaxis given her history of thrombosis; and (3) the impact of age on ovarian reserve. Given the current lack of definitive evidence-based clinical benefit for the removal of an intramural fibroid, after weighing up the risks and limited likely benefit of surgery versus the possible impact on assisted conception outcomes, the couple declined myomectomy initially and opted to proceed to in vitro fertilization (IVF) treatment.

In view of the past history of pulmonary embolism, she was prescribed prophylactic enoxaparin 40 mg daily during IVF treatment, to be continued during pregnancy and postnatally.

Outcome

The couple underwent two cycles of IVF, responding well to 225 IU of FSH in an antagonist cycle. In the first cycle, she had nine eggs retrieved of which six fertilized. In the second cycle, six eggs were retrieved of which five fertilized. On both occasions, she had two embryos transferred but no embryos were suitable for freezing. Neither cycle resulted in a pregnancy. After further discussions, she elected to undergo laparoscopic myomectomy during which two fibroids (10 cm and 2 cm) were removed from the posterior wall. During surgery, it was found that the fibroids were immediately subendometrial although the endometrium had not been breached. She underwent a third cycle of IVF 6 months postoperatively, and this resulted in an ongoing pregnancy and healthy live birth at term.

General remarks

Uterine fibroids occur in up to 30% of women of reproductive age. Most women affected with fibroids are fertile. The evidence regarding the effect of fibroids on fertility depends mainly on the type of fibroid (submucous, intramural, or subserous) and this has been extensively reviewed in several studies [1, 2, 3]. Current observational data suggest the presence of a detrimental effect on fertility of submucous fibroids, while subserous fibroids seem to have little effect. The evidence regarding intramural fibroids is less conclusive and there is no clear consensus regarding the effect of the removal of fibroids on fertility outcomes. A recent Cochrane review [4] concluded that there is currently insufficient evidence from randomized controlled trials (RCTs) to evaluate the role of myomectomy in improving fertility. The only RCT in this review [5] concluded that there was no evidence of benefit of myomectomy for any type of fibroids on clinical pregnancy rate. The management of a couple presenting with uterine fibroids therefore continues to pose a challenge to the practicing fertility specialist. While it is unclear whether or not removal of the fibroids contributed to her achieving a pregnancy in the first postoperative IVF cycle, adequate counseling, thorough pretreatment assessment, and adopting a pragmatic management strategy structured around the patient's progress are likely to have contributed to the optimal management of this couple.

References

1. Klatsky PC, Tran ND, Caughey AB, Fujimoto VY. Fibroids and reproductive outcomes: a systematic literature review from conception to delivery. *Am J Obstet Gynecol* 2008; **198**: 357–66.

2. Metwally M, Farquhar CM, Li TC. Is another meta-analysis on the effects of intramural fibroids on reproductive outcomes needed? *Reprod Biomed Online* 2011; **23**(1): 2–14.

3. Sunkara SK, Khairy M, El-Toukhy T, Khalaf Y, Coomarasamy A. The effect of intramural fibroids without uterine cavity involvement on the outcome of IVF treatment: a systematic review and meta-analysis. *Hum Reprod* 2010; **25**: 418–29.

4. Metwally M, Cheong YC, Horne AW. Surgical treatment of fibroids for subfertility. *Cochrane Database Syst Rev* 2012; (3): CD003857. DOI: 10.1002/14651858.CD003857.pub2.

5. Casini ML, Rossi F, Agostini R, Unfer V. Effect of the position of fibroids on fertility. *Gynecol Endocrinol* 2006 ;**22**(2): 106–9.

Chapter

34

A patient with factor XI deficiency and immune thrombocytopenia

Hammed A. Tijani and Ying Cheong

Clinical fertility history

A 39-year-old police officer presented with a 3-year history of primary subfertility. At the age of 19, she had undergone a left oophorectomy for the removal of a dermoid cyst; this was complicated by intraoperative bleeding requiring blood transfusion. She was later diagnosed with immune thrombocytopenia (ITP) but had never required any treatment for this bleeding disorder. Her periods were heavy but regular. Her partner was fit and well.

General medical, family, and social history

The couple did not smoke or drink alcohol. There was no significant medical history in the family.

Examination findings

The physical examination was unremarkable.

Fertility investigations

The hormone profile was normal. She was rubella immune and chlamydia testing revealed no active infection. Hysterosalpingo-contrast-sonography (Hycosy) showed that she had a bulky retroverted uterus with multiple subserosal fibroids and a 3.5 cm intracavitary fibroid (Type 1) indenting the uterine cavity. Both fallopian tubes were noted to be patent.

Other clinical investigations

The full blood count was essentially normal except for the platelet count that was 79 000/dL (normal 150 000–400 000/dL) due to chronic ITP. She had a mildly prolonged APTT and further hematological investigations confirmed the additional diagnosis of mild factor XI deficiency.

Diagnosis

Primary subfertility associated with uterine fibroids, chronic immune thrombocytopenia, and mild factor X1 deficiency.

Action plan

Given the patient's age and the duration of subfertility, the patient elected to undergo IVF.

Management of bleeding disorder preoperatively

Given the presence of fibroid disrupting the endometrial cavity, surgery was recommended to improve her chances of conception prior to IVF. The pre operative management of her bleeding disorder agreed between the gynecological surgeon and the hematologist was as follows:

1. Dexamethasone treatment for 4 days prior to surgery.
2. Oral tranexamic acid 1 g immediately pre op, to be continued 8-hourly afterwards for a week.
3. Fresh frozen plasma should be available for transfusion in case of intra- or postoperative bleeding.
4. A combination of compression stockings with early mobilization rather than enoxaparin was recommended for thromboprophylaxis.

The patient had a preoperative platelet count of 80 000/dL, which was deemed adequate to proceed with surgery. The patient underwent an uneventful hysteroscopic myomectomy where a 3 cm Type 1 fundal fibroid (encroaching the uterine cavity) was resected.

Outcome

Following her myomectomy, she went on to have IVF treatment using the antagonist protocol with 225 units of recombinant FSH. Eighteen eggs were collected; nine were fertilized, and two embryos were transferred and two embryos were frozen.

Management of bleeding disorder during egg collection

Because her platelet count was over 50 000/dL, the patient was advised to take tranexamic acid prior to oocyte retrieval and for 24 h afterwards.

General remarks

The successful management of this patient required a multidisciplinary approach involving the fertility specialist, the surgeon, and the hematologist.

Inherited factor XI deficiency

Also called hemophilia C or Rosenthal syndrome, this is an uncommon autosomal recessive disorder. It is characterized by a more variable bleeding tendency than hemophilia A or B.

Patients with severe factor XI (FXI) deficiency (plasma FXI activity <15 U/dL) do not usually bleed spontaneously but may do so when they suffer excessive injury or undergo surgery. In patients with milder defects (plasma FXI 15–60 U/dL), bleeding is, however, difficult to predict because it correlates poorly with FXI levels, thus making the clinical management of such patients particularly challenging [1]. Bleeding is more likely when trauma involves tissues rich in fibrinolytic activity such as urogenital and oral mucosal area. Patients with FXI deficiency do not need treatment or prophylaxis for routine functions or activities. However, they do need treatment prior to surgery.

For severe deficiency, replacement therapy with virally inactivated fresh frozen plasma (FFP) or FXI concentrates is the mainstay of treatment [1]. Antifibrinolytic agents such as tranexamic acid have been useful for the management of mild cases of Factor XI deficiency and for minor surgical procedures. The treatment usually begins before the procedure and continues for an additional week. Occasionally, desmopressin (DDAVP), a synthetic analog of the natural antidiuretic hormone vasopressin, plasma, prothrombin complex concentrates, and recombinant activated factor VII have also been used. Unless needed for another medical indication, patients with factor XI deficiency should avoid aspirin and NSAIDs.

The management of immune thrombocytopenia (ITP)

Management of ITP is dependent on the patient's platelet level and the type of procedure that is being undertaken. Intraoperative bleeding complications are unusual if the platelet count is greater than 50 000/dL. Steroids (prednisolone) are usually the first-line therapy in stable patients. An increase in platelet count is observed usually within 3–5 days. Intravenous immunoglobulin (IVIG) can be utilized in patients who do not respond to prednisone.

Reference

1. Franchini M, Manzato F, Salvagno GL, Montagnana M, Lippi G. The use of desmopressin in congenital factor XI deficiency: a systematic review. *Ann Hematol* 2009; **88**(10): 931–5.

Further reading

Howman RA, Barr AL, Shand AW, Dickinson JE. Antenatal intravenous immunoglobulin in chronic immune thrombocytopenic purpura: case report and literature review. *Fetal Diagn Ther* 2009; **25**(1): 93–7.

Nelson SM, Greer IA. The patient at risk from thrombosis and bleeding disorders. In: Macklon N *et al.* (eds.) *Textbook of Periconceptional Medicine*. London: Informa; 2009.

Abnormal cavity; abnormal fertility?

Jenneke C. Kasius

Clinical fertility history

A 39-year-old Nigerian woman was admitted with an 18-month history of secondary infertility. Seven years previously while living in Nigeria she had undergone a pregnancy termination at 12 weeks of gestation. She had moved to Europe 5 months before presentation, and then met her current partner who was 37 years old and had one 4-year-old child from a former relationship. She described a regular menstrual cycle and self ovulation testing had shown positive results.

General medical, family, and social history

Both the woman and her partner were healthy. The woman worked as a nurse, and her partner was a physiotherapist. They do not suffer from any chronic conditions. Besides the previous surgical termination of pregnancy, she had not undergone any other operative procedures. The couple did not report using any medication, tobacco, or alcohol. She had no contact with her relatives. Her partner's family history was unremarkable.

Examination findings

The woman had a BMI of 26 kg/m^2, and gynecological examination revealed no abnormalities.

Fertility investigations

Transvaginal ultrasound (TVS) revealed an intrauterine structure suggestive of a small intracavitary polyp. Endocrine investigation showed a FSH of 11 IU/L on cycle day 4, The *Chlamydia* antibody titer was negative. Hysterosalpingography (HSG) showed a normal uterine cavity and tubal patency.

Other clinical investigations

At hysteroscopy, a normal, symmetrical-shaped uterine cavity was seen. On the posterior wall of the uterine fundus a small polyp of 1.0 cm was detected. The lesion was excised without complication using hysteroscopic scissors. Histological investigation of the removed tissue confirmed the diagnosis of a benign endometrial polyp.

Diagnosis

Primary infertility of unexplained origin other than the possible contribution of an endometrial polyp.

Action plan

Regular IVF was scheduled 3 months after the hysteroscopy.

Outcome

The woman conceived spontaneously just before the start of the IVF treatment. Unfortunately, she had a spontaneous miscarriage at 5 weeks of gestation. Within the year after the miscarriage, three IVF cycles were performed, from which she did not conceive.

General remarks

Intrauterine polyps, myomata, and adhesions are the most frequently reported intrauterine abnormalities. They are assumed to negatively interfere with the chance of conceiving. In the IVF population, a distinction must be made between patients with abnormalities which may impact on outcome of treatment and those without. Suspicion of intrauterine abnormalities can arise on the basis of symptoms, such as reported menstruation disorders, or abnormal findings at fertility investigation by TVS or hysterosalpingography. Treatment is generally provided by means of (outpatient) hysteroscopy.

In populations suspected of intrauterine polyps, myomata, or adhesions, numerous studies have been performed to investigate the impact of the abnormality on fertility. Most of the studies are retrospective, or compare one group of patients before and after hysteroscopic treatment of the abnormality. The results of these studies are discordant. Moreover, high-quality evidence for the effect of intrauterine abnormalities is sparse. Only the impacts of polypectomy and myomectomy on fertility have been investigated in small randomized controlled trials. Polypectomy appears to increase the chances of conception, both spontaneously and after intrauterine insemination [1]. Two studies have indicated that the removal of subserosal fibroids may be beneficial, with borderline statistical significance [2, 3].

The prevalence of intrauterine abnormalities in asymptomatic infertile patients has been reported to be 11–45% [4, 5, 6]. So far, the best available evidence on the impact of minor abnormalities at hysteroscopy in patients with a normal TVS or HSG consists of two RCTs. In a population with ≥2 failed IVF cycles a subsequent pregnancy rate of 9–13% was reported when hysteroscopy was performed and abnormalities were treated [3, 7, 8].

In conclusion, there appears to be some benefit for fertility outcomes when intrauterine abnormalities are sought and treated hysteroscopically. However, high-quality evidence that confirms this positive effect is still required before routine treatment of and screening for abnormalities by hysteroscopy prior IVF can be recommended [9, 10]. Until then, the management of the (un)suspected intrauterine abnormalities should be individualized for each patient and each abnormality.

References

1. Pérez-Medina T, Bajo-Arenas J, Salazar F, Redondo T, Sanfrutos L, Alvarez P et al. Endometrial polyps and their implication in the pregnancy rates of patients undergoing intrauterine insemination: a prospective, randomized study. *Hum Reprod* 2005; **20**(6): 1632–5.

2. Bosteels J, Weyers S, Puttemans P, Panayotidis C, Herendael van HB, Gomel V et al. The effectiveness of hysteroscopy in improving pregnancy rates in subfertile women without other gynecological symptoms: a systematic review. *Hum Reprod Update* 2010; **16**(1): 1–11.

3. Casini ML, Rossi F, Agostini R, Unfer V. Effect of the position of fibroids on fertility. *Gynecol Endocrinol* 2006; **22**(2): 106–9.

4. Balmaceda JP, Ciuffardi I. Hysteroscopy and assisted reproductive technology. *Obstet Gynecol Clin North Am* 1995; **22**: 507–18.

5. Fatemi HM, Kasius JC, Timmermans A, Disseldorp van J, Fauser BC, Devroey P *et al.* Prevalence of unsuspected uterine cavity abnormalities diagnosed by office hysteroscopy prior to in vitro fertilization. *Hum Reprod* 2010; **25**(8): 1959–65.

6. Hinckley MD, Milki AA. 1000 office-based hysteroscopies prior to in vitro fertilization: feasibility and findings. *JSLS* 2004; **8**(2): 103–7.

7. Demirol A, Gurgan T. Effect of treatment of intrauterine pathologies with office hysteroscopy in patients with recurrent IVF failure. *Reprod Biomed Online* 2004; **8**(5): 590–4.

8. Rama Raju GA, Shashi KG, Krishna KM, Prakash GJ, Madan K. Assessment of uterine cavity by hysteroscopy in assisted reproduction programme and its influence on pregnancy outcome. *Arch Gynecol Obstet* 2006; **274**(3): 160–4.

9. El-Toukhy T, Campo R, Sunkara SK, Khalaf Y, Coomarasamy A. A multi-centre randomised controlled study of pre-IVF outpatient hysteroscopy in women with recurrent IVF implantation failure: Trial of Outpatient Hysteroscopy-[TROPHY] in IVF. *Reprod Health* 2009; **6**: 20.

10. Smit JG, Kasius JC, Eijkemans MJ, Koks CA, Van Golde R, Oosterhuis JG *et al.* The inSIGHT study: costs and effects of routine hysteroscopy prior to a first IVF treatment cycle. A randomised controlled trial. *BMC Womens Health* 2012; **12**: 22.

A male partner with 'flu

Elisabeth Carlsen

Clinical fertility history

A 31-year-old woman and her 34-year-old husband with a 3-year history of primary infertility were referred for treatment using IVF. They had previously been treated with three cycles of intrauterine insemination using the husband's sperm. The numbers of progressive motile sperms inseminated in each cycle had been 4.2 million, 5.1 million, and 3.7 million, respectively, but no conception had occurred. The patient underwent stimulation for IVF with r-FSH after pituitary down-regulation and developed 10 follicles. However, on the day of oocyte pick-up, two successive semen samples revealed azoospermia.

General medical, family, and social history

The woman was a healthy nonsmoking clerk. She had an uneventful past medical history except for surgery for appendicitis as a child. She had taken oral contraceptives from age 18 until 28 years and reported regular menstrual cycles of 27–29 days over the preceding 2½ years. She had never suffered any sexually transmitted disease, and was taking no medication.

Her husband was a healthy nonsmoking sales manager. He had no history of cryptorchidism, orchitis, previous sexually transmitted diseases, or urogenital surgery. He was taking no medication and denied using anabolic steroids.

Examination findings

The woman's clinical examination was normal and she had a BMI of 21 kg/m². She tested negative for active *Chlamydia trachomatis*. An ultrasound scan was performed on cycle day 8 and a normal uterus was visualized with a three-layered endometrium measuring 5.4 mm in thickness. Both ovaries were located close to the vaginal vault. In all, 18 antral follicles were counted. Her husband had a BMI of 23 kg/m² and demonstrated normal virilization, with no gynecomastia. Both testicles were located in the scrotum, measuring by palpation 15 mL on the right side and 12 mL on the left side. There was no sign of varicocele or hydrocele. A normal epididymis and ductus deferens was palpated on each side. An ultrasound scan of the testicles showed a regular pattern without calcifications or tumors.

Fertility investigations

Female: A hysterosalpingogram performed previously had shown normal tubal patency. Serum progesterone on cycle day 22 was 42 nmol/L (5.3–86 nmol/L). Endocrine profile on CD 2 showed no evidence of ovarian or thyroid dysfunction.

Table 36.1 Partner's semen parameters

Parameter	Semen sample number		Reference[a]
	1	2	
Duration of abstinence (days)	2	3	
Semen volume (mL)	1.5	1.5	1.5 (1.4–1.7)
Sperm concentration (million/mL)	39	61	15 (12–16)
Total motility (%)	66	59	40 (38–42)
Progressive motility (%)	32	28	32 (31–34)
Sperm morphology normal (%)	9	10	4 (3.0–4.0)

[a] Lower reference limits (5th centiles and their 95% confidence intervals) for semen characteristics.

Male: Serum endocrine investigations revealed the following results: LH 2.4 IU/L (1.7–8.6 IU/L), FSH 5.4 IU/L (<11 IU/L), inhibin B 217 pg/mL (50–325 pg/mL), total testosterone 23.4 nmol/L (7.6–31 nmol/L), sex hormone-binding globulin 32 nmol/L (10–37 nmol/L), prolactin 125 mIU/L (60–250 mIU/L). Karyotype analysis was normal 46,XY.

Two semen samples had been performed 2 and 1½ years previously as part of the initial workup. Semen analysis was performed according to the WHO manual 2010 using strict criteria for morphology [1].

Semen parameters were as listed in Table 36.1.

Duration of abstinence was 2–7 days in the material on which the reference limits were based [1]. Usually a duration of abstinence of 2–3 days is recommended for semen analysis.

A semen sample had been analyzed 2 weeks prior to the IVF attempt, showing reduced sperm concentration of 12 mill/mL and total motility of 38%, and only 5% morphologically normal spermatozoa.

Diagnosis

The sudden deterioration in semen parameters prompted an interview and further physical examination of her partner. There was a normal physical examination and ultrasound scan of the testicles. There had been no change in lifestyle factors and no medications; however, he reported having suffered an influenza infection with high fever (39–40°C) for 5 days, commencing 3 weeks prior to the IVF attempt.

Action plan

It was suspected that the fever associated with influenza was responsible for the azoospermia, and a second semen sample 1½ months later was planned prior to a further IVF attempt.

Outcome

A semen sample analyzed 2½ months after the influenza showed normalization of semen quality as follows: duration of abstinence 3 days; semen volume 1.5 mL; sperm concentration 38 million/mL; total motility 64%; progressive motility 31%; and sperm morphology normal 9%. A second IVF attempt was subsequently undertaken, resulting in normal fertilization.

General remarks

The case illustrates the detrimental effect of fever on semen parameters. A number of published case studies have reported the negative impact of fever on semen parameters. In an early report, a marked decrease in sperm concentration, motility, and morphology arose in association with fever secondary to chickenpox and pneumonia [2]. Sperm concentration did not recover until 60 days after normalization of the temperature, whereas motility and morphology recovered after 30 days. This time-course is in accordance with the results obtained in a larger study of 27 young men being followed with monthly semen samples for 16 months during which 15 experienced a febrile episode [3]. In this study it was demonstrated that sperm concentration decreased on average by 33% and sperm motility and morphology by 20% and 7% respectively during a time period from 8 to 30 days after the febrile event. It was also seen that sperm concentration did not recover until almost 60 days after the febrile event. The sperm parameters were increasingly affected with increasing number of days of fever. One of the subjects who recorded fever with temperature rise to 39–40°C for 6 days demonstrated a decrease in sperm concentration of 95%. Notably, semen parameters were not significantly affected for the first 8 days following initiation of febrile disease. The changes in semen parameters due to fever can be related to the different phases of the spermatogenic cycle: mitotic divisions of spermatogonia, meiotic divisions of spermatocytes, spermiogenesis (postmeiotic phase), and sperm maturation in the epididymis. Sperm concentration appears to be significantly affected during both meiosis and spermiogenesis, whereas sperm motility and morphology are primarily affected during spermiogenesis. A similar effect of fever on sperm concentration and motility has been demonstrated more recently in a fertile donor with temperature increase to 39–40°C [4]. In this study it was also found that fever caused a temporary increase in sperm DNA fragmentation.

References

1. World Health Organization. Examination and Processing of Human Semen. 5th ed. Geneva: WHO; 2010.

2. MacLeod J. Effect of chickenpox and of pneumonia on semen quality. *Fertil Steril* 1951; **2**: 523–33.

3. Carlsen E, Andersson A-M, Petersen JH, Skakkebæk NE. History of febrile illness and variation in semen quality. *Hum Reprod* 2003; **18**: 2089–92.

4. Sergerie M, Mieusset R, Croute F, Daudin M, Bujan L. High risk of temporary alteration of semen parameters after recent acute febrile illness. *Fertil Steril* 2007; **88**: 970.e1–7.

Selecting the day of triggering final oocyte maturation when follicle growth is asynchronous

E. Papanikolaou

Clinical fertility history

A 35-year-old woman presented with a 2-year history of primary infertility. She had under-gone laparoscopic excision of bilateral endometriomas at the age of 25 years. She had refused earlier referral, assuming her fertility normal.

General medical, family, and social history

Her medical history was free and she was not a smoker. Her mother gave birth after spon-taneous conception to her and her brother.

Examination findings

Physical examination revealed a woman weighing 52 kg of height 167 cm. Gynecological examination was negative. No signs of thyroid gland abnormalities were present.

Fertility investigations

Intravaginal ultrasound revealed a normal uterus, low antral follicle count in both ovaries, and signs of hydrosalpinx at the left adnexa. Her endocrine profile on cycle day 3 was normal with FSH of 7.2m IU/mL. She underwent hysterosalpingography, which revealed that both tubes were blocked with signs of hydrosalpinx. AMH was measured and was 0.9 ng/mL. The rest of the blood tests were normal.

Her husband's sperm was normal with more than 120 million total sperm count and more than 50% motility after 1 hour.

Other clinical investigations

She underwent laparoscopy, where both tubes were removed. At the same time hysteroscopy showed a small septum, which was excised.

Diagnosis

IVF was proposed and the patient started down-regulation with buserelin in a long protocol. Three weeks after down-regulation and one after her period, 300 IU of rec-FSH was initiated.

Action plan

At day 8 of stimulation she already had two follicles of 20 mm and four medium follicles of 14–15 mm. Her estradiol was 900 pg/mL, but progesterone was 2.4 ng/mL. Since her progesterone was prematurely raised [1], we decided that no fresh embryo-transfer would take place. We therefore decided to proceed with two more days in stimulation in order to retrieve more oocytes than the two dominant. Two days later the four follicles were 17–19 mm and the two leading follicles had increased to 24–25 mm. The progesterone value was 6.3 ng/mL. Recombinant hCG 250 µg was administered and 36 hours later four oocytes were retrieved (none from the large follicles). Conventional IVF was applied and three zygotes were produced. On day 3 in the luteal phase three top-quality embryos were cryopreserved.

Outcome

After the three frozen embryos were thawed, two survived 100% at the 8-cell stage with <10% fragmentation. In an estrogen substitution cycle, the two embryos were transferred on day 4 after the progesterone supplementation. A twin pregnancy occurred. The patient delivered at 34 weeks, and two healthy boys were born.

General remarks

A common dilemma encountered in IVF practice is when to trigger ovulation in the case that one or two follicles are already dominant and the rest are following. The solution is easy if the patient is a normo-responder and the follicles that follow are in the majority: ignore the dominant, aiming for the rest of the follicles. However, if the patient is a poor responder and has one or two follicles advanced more than 2 days in diameter, and the rest following are three or four, then the decision is difficult and even controversial. We suggest looking at the progesterone levels [2]. If progesterone is normal (<1.5 ng/mL) and there are two follicles ready, whereas the rest are three or even four, it might be better to trigger ovulation and to go for the two dominant follicles. On the other hand, if progesterone is rising, endometrial receptivity might decrease [3, 4] and there is also the risk of not finding the dominant oocytes, then it might be better to go for the rest of the follicles, to freeze them all, and later to transfer in a substitute cycle, or even better in a natural cycle retrieving the one dominant follicle. The other option is to cancel the cycle.

References

1. Papanikolaou EG, Pados G, Grimbizis G, Bili E, Kyriazi L, Polyzos NP, Humaidan P, Tournaye H, Tarlatzis B. GnRH-agonist versus GnRH-antagonist IVF cycles: is the reproductive outcome affected by the incidence of progesterone elevation on the day of HCG triggering? A randomized prospective study. *Hum Reprod* 2012; 27: 1822–8.

2. Papanikolaou EG, Kolibianakis EM, Pozzobon C, Tank P, Tournaye H, Bourgain C, Van Steirteghem A, Devroey P. Progesterone rise on the day of human chorionic gonadotropin administration impairs pregnancy outcome in day 3 single-embryo transfer, while it has no effect on day 5 single blastocyst transfer. *Fertil Steril* 2009; 91: 949–52.

3. Van Vaerenbergh I, Fatemi HM, Blockeel C, Van Lommel L, In't Veld P, Schuit F, Kolibianakis EM, Devroey P, Bourgain C. Progesterone rise on HCG day in GnRH antagonist/rFSH stimulated cycles affects endometrial gene expression. *Reprod Biomed Online* 2011; 22: 263–71.

4. Bosch E, Labarta E, Crespo J, Simón C, Remohí J, Jenkins J, Pellicer A. Circulating progesterone levels and ongoing pregnancy rates in controlled ovarian stimulation cycles for in vitro fertilization: analysis of over 4000 cycles. *Hum Reprod* 2010; 25: 2092–100.

Late-onset ovarian hyperstimulation syndrome (OHSS)

38

Leo Doherty and Saioa Torrealday

Case presentation

A 34-year-old woman, gravida 0 with primary infertility of 3 years duration, presented to our center requesting fertility treatment for anovulation. Her medical and surgical histories were negative. Her family history was noncontributory. Her gynecological history was notable for menarche at age 10 years, and irregular menstrual cycles occurring every 35–60 days, with menses 4–8 days in duration. She denied any history of dysmenorrhea, abnormal Pap smears, or sexually transmitted diseases. On physical examination, her BMI was 25 kg/m². She had hirsutism on the sideburns and chin area. She did not exhibit acanthosis nigricans or clitoromegaly. Pelvic examination was within normal limits. Transvaginal ultrasonography revealed a normal appearing uterus. Ovaries did not appear polycystic in appearance and the antral follicle count was 18. Her cycle day 3 follicle stimulating-hormone (FSH) was 5.4 mIU/mL, estradiol (E2) 52 pg/mL, and luteinizing hormone (LH) 4.7 mIU/mL.

Her partner was a 38-year-old man with no significant past medical history. He was on no medications and had never fathered any children. His workup consisted of a normal semen analysis and infectious disease evaluation.

Fertility treatment history

After three cycles of clomiphene citrate and intrauterine insemination (IUI) and one cycle of injectable gonadotropin and IUI without success, the decision was made to proceed with in vitro fertilization (IVF).

The IVF stimulation protocol was preceded by oral contraceptive pills overlapping with GnRHa to achieve pituitary down-regulation. Ovarian stimulation was then carried out with 150 IU/day of recombinant human FSH (Gonal-F, EMD Serono) for 8 days, followed by 112.5 IU for 1 day, then 75 IU for 1 day. After a total of 11 days of stimulation, 250 μg of recombinant human hCG (Ovidrel, Merck Serono) was administered. At that time, E2 was 5811 pg/mL. She had 12 follicles ≥18 mm and 24 follicles ≥14 mm. At 36 hours after hCG administration, transvaginal oocyte retrieval yielded 21 oocytes. On day 5, two high-quality embryos were transferred. Ten days after transfer, serum β-hCG was measured at 204 mIU/mL.

Subsequent presentation #1

Forty-eight hours after her initial pregnancy test (12 days after her embryo transfer), the patient presented for evaluation of sharp abdominal pain, which was worsened by eating and while supine. She also noted increasing abdominal distention and weight gain for the preceding 48 hours. She had self-reduced her oral intake due to worsening of her pain after eating. She denied any decrease in urinary output, shortness of breath, or chest pain.

On examination, she was afebrile and her blood pressure, respiratory rate and oxygen saturation were within normal limits. Exam was notable for an elevated pulse rate of 117/min. Her weight was 4 kg greater than it had been before the start of her IVF cycle. She was in no acute distress. Cardiac and pulmonary examinations were within normal limits. Abdominal examination revealed a soft, slightly distended abdomen that was mildly tender to palpation diffusely without rebound or guarding. Her extremities were nontender and nonedematous. Pelvic examination was deferred.

Transvaginal ultrasound showed a normal-appearing uterus with a thickened endometrial stripe. The right ovary was enlarged and multicystic, measuring 7.1 × 4.9 × 4.9 cm. The left ovary was also enlarged and multicystic, measuring 6.2 × 5.7 × 6.6 cm. Free fluid was present throughout the pelvis and the largest measurable pocket of fluid was 6.1 × 3 cm.

Laboratory assessment included complete blood count (CBC), complete metabolic panel (CMP), prothrombin time/International Normalized Ratio (PT/INR), and partial thromboplastin time (PTT). CBC was notable for a white blood cell (WBC) count of $14.6 \times 10^3/\mu L$, hemoglobin of 13.5 g/dL, hematocrit of 39.6%, and platelet count of 462×1000/mL. Sodium was 134 mmol/L, potassium 3.9 mmol/L, and creatinine 0.8 mg/dL. Transaminases (ALT, AST) were normal. Repeat serum β-hCG was 427 mIU/mL.

At this time, the clinical presentation was consistent with grade I–II (mild-moderate) ovarian hyperstimulation syndrome (OHSS). She was counseled to monitor her fluid balance by recording her oral fluid intake and urinary output. She was also instructed to check her weight daily. She was discharged to home with a plan for repeat serum β-hCG and evaluation in 48 hours.

Subsequent presentation #2

Ninety-six hours after her initial pregnancy test (14 days after embryo transfer) she returned for repeat evaluation. Her abdominal discomfort and distention were slightly worse than they had been 48 hours previously. She complained of fatigue and mild dyspnea while supine. She denied chest pain and dyspnea when upright.

She continued to be mildly tachycardic with a pulse of 102/min. Oxygen saturation was 99% on room air. Her weight was 1 kg greater than it had been 48 hours prior (a total weight gain of 5 kg). Pulmonary examination revealed decreased breath sounds at the bases bilaterally. Cardiac examination was within normal limits. Results of abdominal and extremity examinations were unchanged. Transvaginal ultrasonography showed ovarian sizes that were stable compared to the ultrasound 48 hours prior; however, the degree of pelvic ascites was increased. The maximal pocket of ascites in the posterior cul-de-sac was 10 cm × 8 cm.

Repeat laboratory assessment revealed the following: WBC $10.8 \times 10^3/\mu L$, hemoglobin 14 g/dL, hematocrit 42.3%, and platelet count 488×10^3/mL. Sodium was 140 mmol/L, potassium 4.1 mmol/L, and creatinine 0.9 mg/dL. Transaminases were mildly elevated with AST of 74 U/L and ALT of 70 U/L.

At this time, her clinical presentation was consistent with grade II (moderate) OHSS. Given her degree of discomfort and worsening ascites, the decision was made to proceed with transvaginal ultrasound-guided paracentesis (culdocentesis). Nine hundred mL of tea-colored ascites was removed and the patient's symptoms were improved.

Outcome

Her symptoms improved following culdocentesis. Abdominal distention persisted, but with slightly less pain, and her dyspnea resolved. Her weight was unchanged for the remainder of the first trimester. Serum β-hCG measurements were performed serially every 48 hours until they reached 2000 mIU/mL. Transvaginal ultrasound, performed at 5 weeks + 6 days, revealed a dichorionic/diamniotic twin gestation. Transvaginal ultrasounds were performed every 1–2 weeks until 12 weeks. She experienced mild cramping and spotting at 7 weeks, which resolved spontaneously at 11 weeks. At 12 weeks, she was transferred to her referring obstetrician. Her pregnancy was complicated by spontaneous preterm labor at 26 weeks gestation, at which time she was admitted to the antepartum unit. She delivered viable twin girls at 30 weeks via primary cesarean section.

Case summary

A 34-year-old G0 with primary infertility underwent a long-protocol down-regulation IVF cycle, with peak E2 levels of 5811 pg/mL and 21 oocytes retrieved. She had a day five-embryo transfer of two blastocysts. Ten days after transfer (19 days after hCG trigger), she had a positive serum β-hCG and began to have worsening symptoms and clinical and laboratory findings consistent with grade II OHSS. She underwent culdocentesis, and was managed expectantly as an outpatient. She ultimately delivered viable female infants at 30 weeks after presenting at 26 weeks with spontaneous preterm labor.

Discussion of OHSS

Ovarian hyperstimulation syndrome is an iatrogenic complication associated with exogenous gonadotropin administration during assisted reproductive technology (ART) cycles and is rarely seen in patients treated with clomiphene citrate [1]. The syndrome occurs after luteinization of multiple ovarian follicles and is characterized by increased capillary permeability that results in fluid shifts out of the vascular space [2]. Vascular endothelial growth factor (VEGF), secreted by luteinized ovarian follicles, is a vasoactive substance that disrupts the functional integrity of blood vessels and results in fluid shifts [3]. These fluid shifts can result in massive ascites and hypovolemia that lead to hemoconcentration, decreased blood pressure, tachycardia, and end-organ damage. Severe OHSS can cause massive hemoconcentration and intravascular depletion and result in devastating complications, including renal failure, hypovolemic shock, acute respiratory distress syndrome (ARDS), venous thromboembolism, and death.

Because luteinization of ovarian follicles is required for the development of OHSS, symptoms are not seen until after exogenous hCG (which mimics an ovulatory LH surge) or GnRH agonist (used to promote pituitary secretion on endogenous LH) is administered. One of the drawbacks of exogenous hCG administration, compared with stimulation of endogenous LH using GnRH agonists, is its long half-life. Serum hCG levels are detectable up to 14 days after intramuscular administration of exogenous hCG [4]. When GnRH agonists are used to induce an endogenous LH surge, LH levels return to baseline by 36 hours [5].

OHSS exists in two patterns. Early OHSS occurs within 3–7 days of hCG administration and is associated with exaggerated response to gonadotropin stimulation. Women with elevated E2 levels and high numbers of oocytes retrieved are at greater risk for early OHSS. Late OHSS occurs 12–17 days after hCG administration in cycles where pregnancy is achieved.

hCG secreted from implanting trophoblasts acts to stimulate ovarian production of vasoactive substances such as VEGF. Multiple gestations are associated with more severe presentation of late OHSS, presumably due to higher hCG levels. Late OHSS is often more severe than early OHSS. The sustained production of endogenous hCG after successful embryo implantation likely contributes to the severity of late OHSS.

Management of OHSS varies from institution to institution, but common management themes are universal. Common therapies in the management of OHSS include careful intravenous fluid administration, correction of electrolyte imbalances, thromboprophylaxis with subcutaneous heparin or low-molecular-weight heparin (with substantial hemoconcentration, i.e., hematocrit >45 or 50), and paracentesis (either transabdominal or transvaginal). Outpatient management is possible unless patients exhibit intractable pain, intractable nausea, respiratory compromise, venous thromboembolism, or severe electrolyte abnormalities. While the mainstay of treatment is supportive care, the most successful strategy for management of OHSS is primary prevention. Patients at high risk for OHSS (young age, polycystic ovary syndrome, history of OHSS) should be followed closely and IVF stimulation protocols that decrease the incidence of OHSS (such as those that allow for GnRH agonist triggers) should be considered.

The case described is an excellent example of the time course and clinical findings seen in late-onset OHSS. The patient was not symptomatic between 3 and 7 days after hCG trigger, ruling out early OHSS. She began to experience symptoms 19 days after hCG administration. Her symptoms, examination, and laboratory findings were all consistent with fluid shifting out of the intravascular compartment and into her abdomen. Following supportive care and transvaginal ultrasound-guided paracentesis, her clinical picture improved. Of note, the premature delivery of her twins was not thought to be related to her OHSS.

References

1. Vlahos NF, Gregoriou O. Prevention and management of ovarian hyperstimulation syndrome. *Ann N Y Acad Sci* 2006; **1092**: 247–64.

2. Goldsman MP, Pedram A, Dominguez CE, Ciuffardi I, Levin E, Asch RH. Increased capillary permeability induced by human follicular fluid: a hypothesis for an ovarian origin of the hyperstimulation syndrome. *Fertil Steril* 1995; **63**(2): 268–72.

3. Levin ER, Rosen GF, Cassidenti DL, Yee B, Meldrum D, Wisot A *et al.* Role of vascular endothelial cell growth factor in ovarian hyperstimulation syndrome. *J Clin Invest* 1998; **102**(11):1978–85.

4. Damewood MD, Shen W, Zacur HA, Schlaff WD, Rock JA, Wallach EE. Disappearance of exogenously administered human chorionic gonadotropin. *Fertil Steril* 1989; 52(3): 398–400.

5. Fauser BC, de Jong D, Olivennes F, Wramsby H, Tay C, Itskovitz-Eldor J *et al.* Endocrine profiles after triggering of final oocyte maturation with GnRH agonist after cotreatment with the GnRH antagonist ganirelix during ovarian hyperstimulation for in vitro fertilization. *J Clin Endocrinol Metab* 2002; **87**(2): 709–15.

The patient with recurrent poor embryo quality

Cindy M. P. Duke and Pasquale Patrizio

Case presentation

A 37-year-old gravida 0 woman presented with 4 years of unexplained primary infertility, after completely normal hormonal assessment, hysterosalpingography, and semen analysis. She had previously undergone three failed cycles of intrauterine insemination (IUI) and three cycles of IVF which showed good fertilization (70%) with either conventional insemination or ICSI on cycle day 1. However all three IVF cycles were notable for poor embryo quality following cleavage on cycle day 2, with the majority of embryos displaying irregular blastomeres, many fragments (grade 4–5 embryos), and developmental arrest by cycle day 3. The transfer of two embryos (4 cells – grade 4 and 3 cells – grade 4) in the first cycle did not result in pregnancy and no transfer was carried out in the subsequent two cycles due to extremely poor embryo quality and arrest. How to proceed in this situation was the challenge presented.

The question of embryo quality is a major consideration in any assisted reproduction cycle. Unfortunately, a minority of infertile patients undergoing IVF present a challenge in that cycle after cycle, despite good oocyte yield or sperm quality, they end up with poorly developing or arrested embryos.

Determining embryo quality

Characterization (good versus poor) of embryo development and thus "quality" is largely determined morphologically on the basis of blastomere size and degree of fragmentation using the grading system first described by Veeck and colleagues [1] (Table 39.1). A modified classification system [2] evaluates and scores embryos (grading) based on the number of blastomeres, blastomere morphology, and fragmentation ranging from grade 1 (best) to grade 5 (worst). A poor-quality embryo can be defined as an embryo with a high degree of fragmentation occupying more than 35% of the cleavage cavity (grades 4 and 5).

Morphological classification is not the most accurate method for selecting embryos competent for implantation. In fact, in many instances, the transfer of morphologically poor-quality embryos has resulted in normal live-born infants. However, when an embryo fails to divide after 24 hours of observation and is scored as grade 4–5, it is considered as arrested and is very unlikely to result in a pregnancy. The principal rationale for not transferring poor-quality embryos has been the belief that they are the result of chromosome aneuploidies or genetic defects of one form or another within the embryo and thus incompatible with growth and implantation.

Biopsy of embryos at either day 3 or day 5 with subsequent pre-implantation genetic screening (PGS) is now commonplace in trying to gather more information on

Table 39.1 Embryo system [1, 2]

Grade 1	Embryo with blastomeres of equal size, no cytoplasmic fragments
Grade 2	Embryo with blastomeres of equal size, minor cytoplasmic fragments or blebs
Grade 3	Embryo with blastomeres of distinctly unequal size; no or few cytoplasmic fragments
Grade 4	Embryo with blastomeres of equal or unequal size; significant cytoplasmic fragmentation
Grade 5	Embryo with few blastomeres of any size; severe or complete fragmentation

Table 39.2 Factors affecting embryo quality

Extrinsic factors	
Culture medium	
Incubator conditions	Temperature Nitrogen Carbon dioxide Oxygen
Embryologist experience/technique	
Endometrial coculture [4]	
Ovarian stimulation protocol	
Fertilization technique	ICSI versus IVF
Intrinsic factors	
Maternal	Age (Increasing age is associated with increased aneuploidy and oocyte cytoplasmic dysfunction [5]) Weight/BMI (increasing BMI has been associated with poorer IVF cycle outcomes [6]) Systemic illness Thyroid dysfunction Dyslipidemia Uncontrolled PCOS Autoimmune disorders Diabetes Karyotype (balanced translocations) Known single gene defects Nutritional status Vitamin D, CoQ_{10}, DHEA, ?DHA Oocyte Cytoplasmic factors ATP, mitochondrial numbers, mitochondrial membrane, mitochondrial DNA, cell death proteins, stress protein ratios, calcium DNA complement (number) and arrangement
Paternal	Karyotype (balanced translocations) Sperm morphology Sperm DNA fragmentation Data is mixed on whether fragmentation by itself without ICSI can affect embryo development Sperm aneuploidies (detected by FISH on sperm) BMI Increasing BMI associated with higher sperm DNA damage [7]
Embryonic	Unknown

the chromosome status of these arrested or poor-quality embryos. Likewise, the recent introduction of time-lapse videocinematography has allowed the continuous observation (photograms every 20 minutes) of embryo morphokinetics and is being used as a criterion to decide which embryo to use for transfer based on strict cleavage times [3]. However, despite the more widespread use of time-lapse and the application of PGS, the data now indicate that some patients, even with chromosomally normal embryos, continue to have poor-quality embryos repeatedly, suggestive of genetic defects. However, these defects are effectively undetectable since we do not know what to look for despite further innovations in screening technologies such as next-generation sequencing. Additionally, with regard to day 3 biopsy, emerging data strongly suggest that genetically abnormal embryos at day 3 are capable of normalizing themselves by day 5. Consequently, a number of intrinsic and extrinsic factors have been implicated and can be further subdivided into maternal, paternal, and embryonic in origin and direct versus indirect. These factors (Table 39.2) play a role in determining the fate of an embryo. However, no one factor has proved to offer a route to a therapeutic panacea. In fact, the etiology largely remains unclear; in so much as any of these factors can be attributable, there are exceptions to the rule for each of them.

Evaluation and management of patients with recurrent poor-quality embryos

The diagnosis of recurrent poor-quality embryos is highly emotionally charged for the patient. This is due, in large part, to the sense of blame that patients place on themselves. Accordingly, careful counseling and appropriate selection of words is paramount. It should be explained to the patient that many factors contribute to this while reviewing the "usual suspects" as listed in Table 39.2. As discussed earlier, there is no clear cut way to predict who will have poor-quality embryos or who will have them repeatedly. However, although evidence to support specific interventions is sparse, the clinician should consider the following steps when such a situation arises:

- Review simulation protocols.
- Review sperm morphology, including DNA fragmentation.
- Gather detailed embryo cleavage information (time lapse, embryoscope).
- Consider early transfer, e.g., postfertilization day 2.
- Embryo co-culture on endometrial cells.
- Consider PGS (even if the embryos arrest and are not suitable for transfer; so as to rule out chromosome aneuploidy).
- Select sperm for ICSI (intracytoplasmic morphologically selected sperm [IMSI], hyaluronic acid [H/A] binding, sperm birefringence).
- Consider donor egg.
- Consider donor sperm.
- Consider referral for mitochondrial DNA transfer (still highly experimental and not allowed in the United States) [8].

References

1. Veeck LL. Preembryo grading and degree of cytoplasmic fragmentation. In: Veeck LL (ed.) *An Atlas of Human Gametes and Conceptuses.* New York: Parthenon; 1999: 40–5.

2. Guelman V. Fertilization and cleavage. In: Patrizio P, Tucker MJ, Guelman V (eds.) *A Color Atlas for Human Assisted Reproduction: Laboratory and Clinical Insights.* Philadelphia: Lippincott, Williams and Wilkins; 2003: 49–69.

3. Chamayou S, Patrizio P, Storaci G, Tomaselli V, Alecci C, Ragolia C, Crescenzo C, Guglielmino A. The use of morphokinetic parameters to select all embryos with full capacity to implant. *J Assist Reprod Genet* 2013; **30** (5): 703–10.

4. Spandorfer SD. Autologous endometrial coculture in patients with a previous history of poor quality embryos. *J Assist Reprod Genet* 2002; **19** (7): 309–12.

5. Jones KT. Meiosis in oocytes: predisposition to aneuploidy and its increased incidence with age. *Hum Reprod Update* 2008; **14**(2): 143–58.

6. Luke B *et al.* The effect of increasing obesity on the response to and outcome of assisted reproductive technology: a national study. *Fertil Steril* 2011; **96**: 820–5.

7. Colaci DS *et al.* Men's body mass index in relation to embryo quality and clinical outcomes in couples undergoing in vitro fertilization. 2012; *Fertil Steril* **98**: 1193–9.

8. Tachibana M *et al.* Exchange of DNA between egg cells may help prevent mitochondrial diseases. *Nature* 2013; **493**: 627–31.

A high progesterone level during ovarian stimulation

Christophe Blockeel and Herman Tournaye

Clinical fertility history

A 31-year-old woman with 2 years of infertility due to ovulation disorders presented at our fertility clinic. After five failed IVF/ICSI treatments in another center, the patient was referred to our clinic for a second opinion. In all of the previous IVF or ICSI attempts, a long protocol with hMG in combination with a nasal GnRH-analog was prescribed. After the first IVF attempt, the patient became pregnant, but unfortunately the pregnancy ended in a miscarriage. Due to poor fertilization, ICSI was chosen instead of conventional IVF for the next attempt. This second attempt resulted in a biochemical pregnancy. The third, fourth, and fifth ICSI attempts remained unsuccessful.

The patient's preliminary examinations (hormonal profile, ultrasound scan, hysterosalpingography) were performed in the other center. The results were all within normal limits, except for the ultrasound scan, which showed PCO-like ovaries. Semen analysis was normal as well as karyotype analysis of both partners. Thyroid function and coagulation tests were checked, but no abnormalities were found. A hysteroscopy was performed, in combination with an endometrial biopsy, and turned out to be normal.

Ovarian stimulation

The patient was prescribed an ICSI treatment using recombinant FSH as ovarian stimulation agent in combination with GnRH antagonist cotreatment. A dose of 150 IU was started on day 2 of the cycle. On day 7 of the cycle (day 6 of the stimulation), subcutaneous administration of the GnRH antagonist ganirelix (Orgalutran) was started at a daily dose of 0.25 mg. Ovarian stimulation was long and the injection for final oocyte maturation was given on the 12th day of stimulation with 10 000 IU of hCG (Pregnyl). The oocyte retrieval, performed under local anesthesia, took place 36 hours after hCG injection. Eleven oocytes were retrieved, of which nine were MII oocytes. Fertilization occurred in 7 of the 9 oocytes, and on day 5 of embryological development two blastocysts were transferred. Other embryos could not be frozen.

The endocrine profile is plotted in Figure 40.1.

The progesterone levels increased progressively from day 9 of the stimulation onward, up to very high values (P = 6.7 ng/mL) on the day of hCG.

Outcome

Even though the endocrine data were available on the day of embryo transfer, her cycle was not cancelled.

Eventually, the patient became pregnant and delivered a healthy baby.

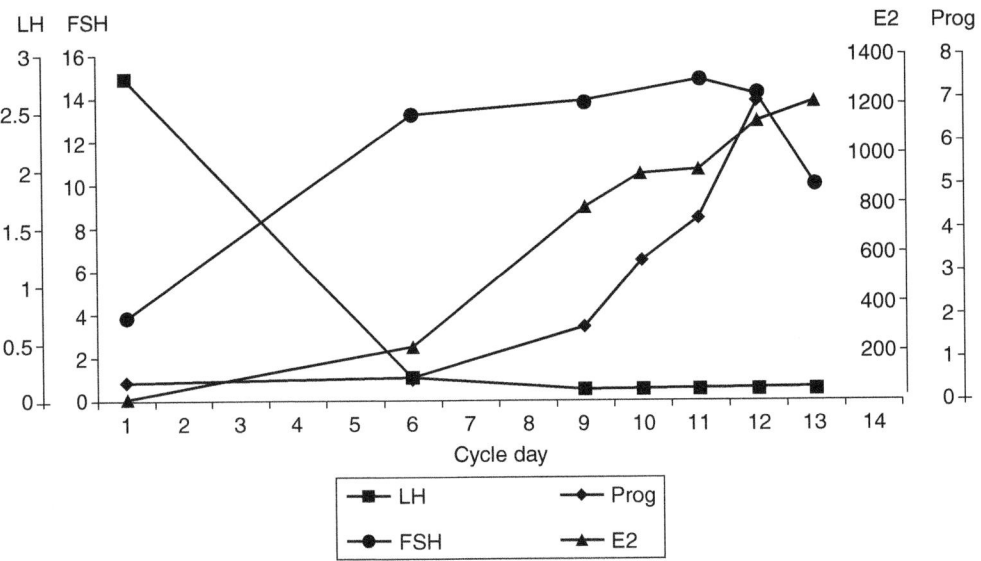

Figure 40.1 Endocrine profile. LH, luteinizing hormone; FSH, follicle-stimulating hormone; Prog, progesterone; E2, estradiol.

Discussion

The effectiveness of in vitro fertilization usually does not exceed 30% per treatment cycle [1] and is further decreased in women older than 36 years of age [2]. Implantation rate depends not only on embryo quality but also on the endometrial receptivity. In this regard, the predictive value of preovulatory hormones for achievement of pregnancy has been evaluated extensively. Progesterone elevation for instance, having an incidence as high as 38% (20–38%) in GnRH antagonist cycles [3, 4], has been subject to a lot of debate because of the negative association between "premature luteinization" and the probability of pregnancy. Conflicting results exist because of different cut-off levels used to define "high" progesterone serum levels [5]. A large retrospective analysis, however, in over 4000 patients, showed that serum progesterone levels above 1.5 ng/mL on the day of hCG administration are associated with a decreased pregnancy rate in GnRH agonists and antagonists [6]. More recent papers in the literature confirm this finding [7, 8]. A systematic review with meta-analysis showed a significantly lower pregnancy rate in the presence of progesterone elevation in patients treated with GnRH antagonists [9]. The mechanism by which these subtle increases in serum progesterone may impact on pregnancy rates is unclear, with data suggesting that elevated progesterone levels may impair endometrial receptivity rather than oocyte quality [10].

Data published in the literature mostly deal with very subtle changes in progesterone levels. To the best of our knowledge, to date no data have been published on cases with extreme elevation of progesterone levels.

In our case, we can speculate that the estradiol concentration caused an extreme increase in ACTH concentrations, stimulating progesterone production from the adrenals.

To conclude, even though there exists a negative association between progesterone elevation on the day of hCG administration (>1.5 ng/mL) and the probability of pregnancy, an extremely high serum progesterone value does not preclude implantation and delivery.

References

1. Andersen AN, Gianaroli L, Felberbaum R, de Mouzon J, Nygren KG. Assisted reproductive technology in Europe, 2001. Results generated from European registers by ESHRE. European IVF-monitoring pro- gramme (EIM). European Society of Human Reproduction and Embryology (ESHRE). *Hum Reprod* 2005; **20**: 1158–76.

2. Stolwijk AM, Wetzels AM, Braat DD. Cumulative probability of achieving an ongoing pregnancy after in-vitro fertilization and intracytoplasmic sperm injection according to a woman's age, subfertility diagnosis and primary or secondary subfertility. *Hum Reprod* 2000; **15**: 203–9.

3. Ubaldi F, Smitz J, Wisanto A, Joris H, Schiettecatte J, Derde MP, Borkham E, Van Steirteghem A, Devroey P. Oocyte and embryo quality as well as pregnancy rate in intracytoplasmic sperm injection are not affected by high follicular phase serum progesterone. *Hum Reprod* 1995; **10**(12): 3091–6.

4. Bosch E, Valencia I, Escudero E, Crespo J, Simón C, Remohí J, Pellicer A. Premature luteinization during gonadotropin-releasing hormone antagonist cycles and its relationship with in vitro fertilization outcome. *Fertil Steril* 2003; **80**(6): 1444–9.

5. Venetis CA, Kolibianakis EM, Papanikolaou E, Bontis J, Devroey P, Tarlatzis BC. Is progesterone elevation on the day of human chorionic gonadotrophin administration associated with the probability of pregnancy in in vitro fertilization? A systematic review and meta-analysis. *Hum Reprod Update* 2007; **13**(4): 343–55.

6. Bosch E, Labarta E, Crespo J, Simón C, Remohí J, Jenkins J, Pellicer A. Circulating progesterone levels and ongoing pregnancy rates in controlled ovarian stimulation cycles for in vitro fertilization: analysis of over 4000 cycles. *Hum Reprod* 2010; **25**(8): 2092–100.

7. Huang R, Fang C, Xu S, Yi Y, Liang X. Premature progesterone rise negatively correlated with live birth rate in IVF cycles with GnRH agonist: an analysis of 2,566 cycles. *Fertil Steril* 2012; **98**(3): 664–70.

8. Xu B, Li Z, Zhang H, Jin L, Li Y, Ai J, Zhu G. Serum progesterone level effects on the outcome of in vitro fertilization in patients with different ovarian response: an analysis of more than 10,000 cycles. *Fertil Steril* 2012; **97**(6): 1321–7.e4.

9. Kolibianakis EM, Venetis CA, Bontis J, Tarlatzis BC. Significantly lower pregnancy rates in the presence of progesterone elevation in patients treated with GnRH antagonists and gonadotrophins: a systematic review and meta-analysis. *Curr Pharm Biotechnol* 2012; **13**(3): 464–70.

10. Fanchin R, Righini C, Olivennes F, Ferreira AL, de Ziegler D, Frydman R. Consequences of premature progesterone elevation on the outcome of in vitro fertilization: insights into a controversy. *Fertil Steril* 1997; **68**(5): 799–805.

Repeated fertilization failure with normal sperm and MII oocytes

Denny Sakkas and Steven Bayer

Background

It has been well established that oocyte quality, and in particular the age of the female, leads to a higher risk of in vitro fertilization failure, miscarriage, and lower live birth rates. When an IVF practitioner is confronted with an infertile couple, a standard evaluation is completed with most of the testing performed on the female partner, including a hystero-salpingogram (HSG) to evaluate the cavity and fallopian tubes and an ovarian reserve assessment. The evaluation of the male is limited to a simple semen analysis, which is only a quantitative assessment of the sperm concentration, motility, and morphology. The WHO has established the normal range for all of these parameters that help with the diagnosis of a male factor. However, the semen analysis is an imprecise test and a previous study confirmed that there is significant overlap of semen parameters between infertile and fertile males [1].

A good percentage of couples (30–40%) have a normal evaluation and fall into the unexplained category. Many of these couples will pursue IVF and in these cases a standard insemination of the eggs is appropriate. Unfortunately, in some cases the couple is faced with the sad news of poor or no fertilization even though oocyte numbers and sperm parameters looked good.

Overall an expected no-fertilization rate of between 1% and 4% will occur after routine insemination of the eggs. Many clinics believe that lack of fertilization can simply be avoided by performing intracytoplasmic sperm injection (ICSI) routinely. In fact the overall utilization rate of ICSI in the United States according to the 2011 Society of Assisted Reproduction Technology Statistics is 66%; this is well over the incidence of male factor infertility, which has been estimated at 30%. This in many cases is a reflex to try to limit the number of failed fertilizations.

Of course for any individual patient complete lack of fertilization is closely related to age and the number of eggs that are available to be inseminated. Assuming a normal fertilization rate of 70%, the lack of fertilization of 3–4 eggs may just be bad luck, whereas the lack of fertilization of 20 eggs clearly has more significance. When examining our own Boston IVF data set we chose to eliminate a possible impact of a female factor and only examined couples in which the female was less than 38 years of age and where more than five oocytes had been collected. The data indicate that, in this patient group, an overall rate of 1.4% failed fertilizations is observed (Table 41.1). This suggests that failed fertilization is more related to a male factor component in approximately 1.4% of cases.

In the state of Massachusetts, insurance companies are mandated to provide coverage for IVF treatment. The approval for ICSI by the insurer is dependent on the parameters of the semen analysis (morphology ≤1% [Strict Morphology]) or when fewer than 3 million

Table 41.1 The number of nondonor cycles presenting with failed fertilization at Boston IVF since January 2010 (a) for all patients with eggs retrieved and (b) where the female partner was less than 38 years of age and had more than five oocytes collected. Couples were treated with either routine IVF or ICS.

	Treatment	Number of cycles	Number of failed fertilizations (%)
(a)	ICSI – All	2838	91 (3.2%)
	IVF– All	3977	155 (3.9%)
	TOTAL – All	6815	246 (3.6%)
(b)	ICSI – <38 years and >5 eggs	1493	20 (1.3%)
	IVF – <38 years and >5 eggs	1967	28 (1.4%)
	TOTAL – <38 years and >5 eggs	3460	48 (1.4%)

total motile sperm are recovered following sperm preparation. From the above patients the failed fertilization rate in routine IVF and ICSI patients, when largely excluding the female factor, is therefore similar (Table 41.1), indicating that the intrinsic sperm characteristics that are responsible for fertilization failure in these couples are not treatable by simply performing ICSI.

Routine semen analysis is a not a qualitative test and therefore fails to provide a real indication whether a couple will experience failed fertilization. To date, no routine semen test can predict whether a couple will experience fertilization failure. The questions therefore remains of how we are to deal with these patients and whether there are any indicators that may provide clues that a particular couple will experience fertilization failure.

Cases of failed fertilization

Two cases are presented (Table 41.2). The first, patient A, underwent routine insemination in three consecutive cycles without achieving a pregnancy. The male produced more than 10 million motile sperm per mL and had normal morphology. In the first cycle a normal fertilization rate of 50% was achieved; however, the second and third cycles saw the fertilization rate drop to 22% and 0% respectively. No attribution could be made in either of these cases to a female factor and at the time of egg retrieval the eggs showed no morphological abnormalities. The case truly indicates that semen values are no indicator of what to expect. Given that the first cycle was below the expected normal fertilization rate of around 65–70%, the question arises whether this patient should have been treated with ICSI directly in the next cycle. Should the first cycle act as a diagnosis for fertilization failure? Unfortunately, the second and third cycles did see an unpredicted precipitous drop in fertilization rate. First cycles which result in a reduced fertilization rate (<50%) could be treated by ICSI for all or a portion of eggs in subsequent cycles to see whether that improves the yield of fertilized embryos (Figure 41.1). Although this treatment could be considered as a proactive way to avoid fertilization failure in subsequent cycles, there are also logistical issues which come into consideration. The greatest of these issues is economic, when the couple cannot afford ICSI, which can cost an additional $1500–2000 in the United States. Some couples also avoid ICSI for safety reasons because of the fear that it may lead to an increased incidence of birth defects.

In Case B (Table 41.2) the couple had already opted to perform ICSI even though semen parameters were normal. In three ICSI cycles only 1 out of a total of 38 eggs was fertilized.

Table 41.2 Two examples of failed fertilization cases where the husband had normal semen values and no female component was diagnosed. The egg morphology appeared normal on the day of egg retrieval

Patient	Age (years)	Number of eggs	Number fertilized	
			IVF (%)	ICSI (%)
A				
Cycle 1	30	16	8 (50%)	
Cycle 2	30	9	2 (22.2%)	
Cycle 3	31	13	0 (0%)	
B				
Cycle 1	34	11		0 (0%)
Cycle 2	34	15		1 (6.6%)
Cycle 3	34	12		0 (0%)

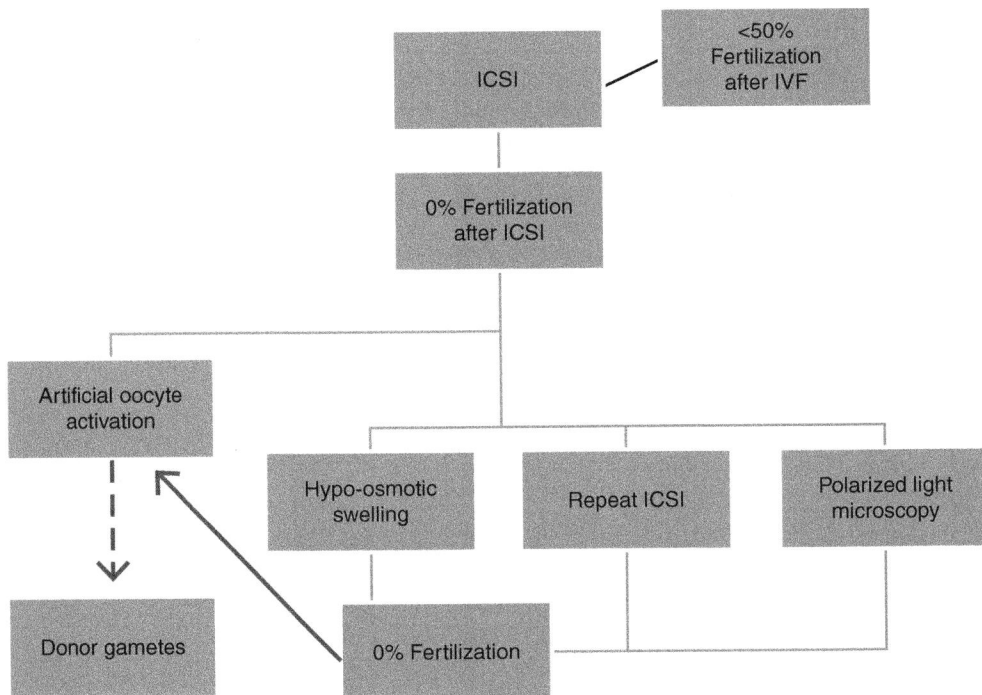

Figure 41.1 Treatment options for patients who have had <50% fertilization in their initial IVF cycle or had failed fertilization after ICSI. A number of techniques can be utilized in subsequent cycles before attempting the more aggressive option of artificial oocyte activation. If failed fertilization persists after three cycles then the couple could be counseled to use donor gametes.

ICSI is believed to be the best treatment option to avoid fertilization failure, but as observed in this case it was of little or no benefit. From Table 41.1 it would appear that approximately 1.3% of cases treated by ICSI are at risk of fertilization failure. In these cases it can be uncertain whether an egg or sperm factor is the one in play.

Methods of improving semen analysis to predict fertilization failure

There are no direct tests to perform on sperm that will predict fertilization failure. A number of diagnostic tests do exist, however, which may provide clues to a defective functionality of the sperm. In the past 20 years numerous tests have been developed for the analysis of sperm nuclear DNA fragmentation (see review [2]). These tests include TdT-mediated dUTP nick-end labeling (TUNEL), the COMET assay, chromomycin A3, in situ nick translation, DBD-FISH (DNA breakage detection–fluorescence in situ hybridization), the sperm chromatin dispersion test (SCD), and the sperm chromatin structure assay (SCSA). Although some data indicate that sperm DNA damage is associated with male infertility and a significantly increased risk of pregnancy loss after IVF and ICSI, no studies have shown a strict correlation with fertilization failure. Indeed, in animal models increasing sperm nuclear DNA damage does not decrease fertilization rates but leads to embryonic and fetal development problems. Other techniques that have been developed to improve semen analysis and sperm selection include hyaluronic acid (HA) binding, deselection of apoptotic sperm, motile sperm organelle morphological examination (MSOME), and the hypo-osmotic swelling (HOS) test [3]. Of these tests, HA binding has been shown to correlate with zona binding [4], but one study examining the use of HA-bound sperm for ICSI in repeated poor-fertilization patients with normal sperm parameters found that it was not helpful [5]. In contrast, the HOS test has been found to provide some important information in normozoospermic male cases with recurrent fertilization failure [6].

Experimental methods of treating fertilization failure

Although a diagnostic method may not exist to predict fertilization failure, some methods of treatment can be used once a patient has experienced one or more fertilization failures after ICSI (Figure 41.1). The methods include artificial oocyte activation, polarization microscopy, and repeated ICSI. In recurrent fertilization failures, artificial oocyte activation can be achieved using Ca^{2+}-ionophore post ICSI to initiate the fertilization process [7]. A number of authors have now reported successful treatment of failed fertilization cases using this technique and it would appear to be the only real option for a case such as Patient B (Table 41.2) to use their own gametes. Polarization microscopy can be used to visualize spindles during ICSI and this may also assist in predicting the optimal time to perform ICSI [8]. Finally, repeat cycles can be treated again by routine ICSI; however, the fertilization rate in most cases remains low if anything.

Conclusion

A diagnostic method to predict fertilization failure does not currently exist. The approach of treating all patients using ICSI will also not eliminate fertilization failures. A proactive treatment plan can, however, be developed for patients who exhibit either poor fertilization or no fertilization in initial treatment cycles (Figure 41.1).

References

1. Guzick DS, Overstreet JW, Factor-Litvak P, Brazil CK, Nakajima ST, Coutifaris C *et al.* Sperm morphology, motility, and concentration in fertile and infertile men. *N Engl J Med* 2001; **345**(19): 1388–93.

2. Sakkas D, Alvarez JG. Sperm DNA fragmentation: mechanisms of origin, impact on reproductive outcome, and analysis. *Fertil Steril* 2010; **93**(4): 1027–36.

3. Henkel R. Sperm preparation: state-of-the-art – physiological aspects and application of advanced sperm preparation methods. *Asian J Androl* 2012; **14**(2): 260–9.

4. Huszar G, Jakab A, Sakkas D, Ozenci CC, Cayli S, Delpiano E *et al.* Fertility testing and ICSI sperm selection by hyaluronic acid binding: clinical and genetic aspects. *Reprod Biomed Online* 2007; **14**(5): 650–63.

5. Choe SA, Tae JC, Shin MY, Kim HJ, Kim CH, Lee JY *et al.* Application of sperm selection using hyaluronic acid binding in intracytoplasmic sperm injection cycles: a sibling oocyte study. *J Korean Med Sci* 2012; **27**(12): 1569–73.

6. Irez T, Usta TA, Zebitay G, Oral E, Senol H, Sahmay S. Evaluation of subgroups of the human sperm hypoosmotic swelling test in normozoospermic male cases with recurrent fertilization failure: a prospective case-controlled study. *Arch Gynecol Obstet* 2013; **287**(4): 797–801.

7. Kashir J, Heindryckx B, Jones C, de SP, Parrington J, Coward K. Oocyte activation, phospholipase C zeta and human infertility. *Hum Reprod Update* 2010; **16**(6): 690–703.

8. Keefe D, Liu L, Wang W, Silva C. Imaging meiotic spindles by polarization light microscopy: principles and applications to IVF. *Reprod Biomed Online* 2003; **7**(1):24–9.

A complete uterine septum

To treat or not to treat?

Jenneke C. Kasius

Clinical fertility history

A 31-year-old woman and her male partner aged 34 presented with secondary infertility of 1 year's duration. She reported one previous pregnancy which had ended in a spontaneous miscarriage at 6 weeks of gestation 1 year previously. She had a regular menstrual cycle of 30 days and described a biphasic temperature curve indicative of ovulatory cycles.

General medical, family, and social history

The couple was generally healthy and neither partner was taking any medication. They did not smoke and used alcohol only on social occasions. Their respective family histories were unremarkable.

Examination findings

General examination of the woman was normal. She has a BMI of 22 kg/m². Gynecological examination showed normal external genitalia, and a normal cervix and vagina at speculum examination. Bimanual examination revealed a mobile, normal-sized uterus and no palpable abnormalities.

Fertility investigations

All investigations were performed on day 3 of the menstrual cycle. Transvaginal sonography (TVS) showed a dense, irregular endometrium of 12 mm thickness. The uterine fundus and both ovaries appeared normal. Her laboratory results were normal, with a FSH of 8.1 IU/L and a negative *Chlamydia* antibody titer.

Semen analysis is normal, with a total motile count of 126 million.

Other clinical investigations

Due to the irregular endometrium on the TVS, saline infusion sonography was performed. This showed a thin septum extending half the length of the uterine cavity. No other abnormalities were visualized.

Diagnosis

A secondary fertility disorder of 1 year of unexplained origin except for the possible impact of the septate uterus.

Action plan

In the absence of a septate uterus, the prognosis to conceive within 1 year of unprotected regular intercourse in unexplained infertility of 1 year's duration would be >50% and justify expectant management. Since no randomized controlled trials (RCTs) are available on the effect of metroplasty on infertility and miscarriage, surgical treatment was not advised.

Outcome

Five months after the visit to the outpatient, the woman reported another spontaneous miscarriage at 5 weeks of gestation. No additional investigations were performed. After a further 4 months she again presented with a spontaneous ongoing pregnancy, which resulted in a vaginal delivery at 35 weeks of gestation after preterm rupture of membranes.

General remarks

During the development of the uterus from the müllerian ducts, congenital anomalies may arise [1]. The septate uterus is the most common congenital anomaly. Uterine anomalies are associated with spontaneous miscarriage and complications during pregnancy and delivery, such as breech presentation, premature labor, and postpartum hemorrhage [2, 3]. The impact of congenital uterine anomalies on fertility continues to be debated.

A number of observational or cohort studies have assessed the effect of metroplasty on female fertility and miscarriage rate. The largest retrospective observational study evaluated the reproductive outcome of 108 patients with unexplained infertility and 138 patients suffering from recurrent abortion [4]. After metroplasty, respectively 57% and 65% of the patients conceived. The miscarriage rate was 19.7% and 34.1%, respectively.

The largest retrospective case–control study compared the chance to conceive after IVF/ICSI before and after metroplasty [5]. These groups were compared to a control group without a septate uterus. The significant difference in pregnancy rate between the group before metroplasty and the control group disappeared after metroplasty.

The one prospective study comparing 44 patients with infertility that was unexplained other than a septate uterus and 132 patients with unexplained infertility without a septate uterus showed a significant increase in live birth rate after metroplasty compared with the control group of patients without a uterine septum [6].

While data from observational and retrospective studies would appear to be consensually in favor of a positive impact of metroplasty in fertility outcomes, there remains a need for well-designed randomized controlled trials to confirm the effect of metroplasty on recurrent miscarriage and infertility [7].

The management of the septate uterus should therefore be based on individual considerations in each patient. Routine metroplasty is certainly not recommended, though it may be considered in patients with a history of adverse pregnancy outcome, prolonged infertility, or more than three miscarriages. The results of an RCT aimed at determining the correct management are awaited [8].

References

1. American Fertility Society. The American Fertility Society classifications of adnexal adhesions, distal tubal occlusions, tubal occlusions secondary to tubal ligations, tubal pregnancies, mullerian anomalies and intrauterine adhesions. *Fertil Steril* 1988; **49**(6): 944–55.

2. Lin PC, Bhatnagar KP, Nettleton GS, Nakajima ST. Female genital anomalies affecting reproduction. *Fertil Steril* 2002; 78(5): 899–915.

3. Taylor E, Gomel V. The uterus and fertility. *Fertil Steril* 2008; 89(1): 1–16.

4. Paradisi R, Barzanti R, Natali F, Battaglia C, Venturoli S. Metroplasty in a large population of women with septate uterus. *J Minim Invasive Gynecol* 2011; 18(4): 449–54.

5. Tomaževič T, Ban-Frangež H, Virant-Klun I, Verdenik I, Požlep B, Vrtačnik-Bokal E. Septate, subseptate and arcuate uterus decrease pregnancy and live birth rates in IVF/ICSI. *Reprod Biomed Online* 2010; 21(5): 700–5.

6. Mollo A, De Franciscis P, Colacurci N, Cobellis L, Perino A, Venezia R *et al.* Hysteroscopic resection of the septum improves the pregnancy rate of women with unexplained infertility: a prospective controlled trial. *Fertil Steril* 2009; 91(6): 2628–31.

7. Kowalik CR, Goddijn M, Emanuel MH, Bongers MY, Spinder T, de Kruif JH *et al.* Metroplasty versus expectant management for women with recurrent miscarriage and a septate uterus. *Cochrane Database Syst Rev* 2011; (6): CD008576.

8. TRUST trial. www.studies-obsgyn.nl/trust NTR 1676. Accessed October 14, 2012.

Chapter 43

Endometritis detected prior to IVF

Jenneke C. Kasius

Clinical fertility history

A couple, both of 38 years, presented to the fertility clinic with a 24-month history of primary infertility. The woman reported a regular cycle of 28 days' duration. They had no history of sexual transmitted disease (STD), nor any symptoms suggestive for STDs, such as intermenstrual or postcoital vaginal bleeding or dyspareunia.

General medical, family, and social history

The woman reported NSAID use for migraine headaches. Neither partner smoked, and both reported drinking one glass of wine a day. Their family histories were negative for both general and fertility disorders.

Examination findings

The woman had a BMI of 23 kg/m². Routine gynecological examination were performed, including inspection of the external genitalia and speculum and bimanual examination. None of the examinations revealed any abnormality.

Fertility investigations

Transvaginal ultrasound was performed and showed a normal uterine shape, endometrium, and myometrium. Also, normal ovaries were visualized and no free fluid in the pelvis was seen. A baseline FSH of 10 IU/L and a weakly positive *Chlamydia* antibody titer were found, and laboratory tests, including *Chlamydia* PCR testing were otherwise normal. Hysterosalpingography revealed normal tubal patency and identified no cavity abnormalities Semen analysis showed a total motile count of 31 million.

Other clinical investigations

Prior to the IVF treatment, a diagnostic hysteroscopy revealed several micropolyps in the uterine cavity, some of which were biopsied. Pathology examination showed the presence of chronic endometritis, as plasma cells were seen in the endometrial stroma.

Diagnosis

Primary infertility disorder lasting 24 months, of unexplained origin other than a possible impact of chronic endometritis.

Action plan

Due to a lack of clarity in the literature regarding the impact of chronic endometritis on fertility, and the efficacy and merit of treatment, it was decided to simply proceed to IVF treatment.

Outcome

After two fresh unsuccessful IVF cycles, pregnancy was achieved from a subsequent cryoembryo transfer. This resulted in the uncomplicated vaginal delivery of a healthy son.

General remarks

Chronic endometritis is a persistent inflammation of the inner lining of the uterine cavity. It is usually asymptomatic and hard to detect by the regular diagnostic tests. Though atypical polyps, edema, or a specific color pattern of the endometrium at hysteroscopy may be suggestive of chronic endometritis, the diagnosis often remains doubtful [1, 2, 3]. The diagnosis is based on a histological detection of plasma cells in an endometrial biopsy. However, the detection of plasma cells can be difficult as plasmacytoid stromal cells may mimic the appearance of plasma cells [4].

While implantation can be considered to be process of physiologic inflammation [5], endotoxins derived from Gram-negative bacteria induce a T-helper-cell 1 reaction and this may result in a hostile intrauterine environment and implantation failure, abortion, or premature labor [6]. However, clinical studies do not clearly demonstrate a negative impact of chronic endometritis on fertility. Often, no causal pathogen can be isolated [7]. The reported prevalence of chronic endometritis in infertile populations varies greatly, between 0.2% and 46% [1, 2, 8, 9]. The literature evaluating the effect on fertility consists of just three studies. In 356 patients with symptoms of pelvic inflammatory disease the pregnancy rate and fertility status did not differ from 258 control patients without endometritis [10]. In a much smaller study, the ongoing pregnancy rate in patients with recurrent IVF failure did not significantly differ between those with and without endometritis [8]. Finally, in a group of asymptomatic, infertile patients the live birth rate was not affected by chronic endometritis, despite antibiotic treatment [9].

In conclusion, based on the current literature, no association between chronic endometritis and infertility has been proven. Furthermore, the positive effect of antibiotic treatment is questionable. Therefore, routine investigation into and treatment of chronic endometritis is not recommended.

References

1. Polisseni F, Banbirra EA, Camargos AF. Detection of chronic endometritis by diagnostic hysteroscopy in asymptomatic infertile patients. *Gynecol Obstet Invest* 2003; 55(4): 205–10.

2. Cicinelli E, Ziegler de D, Nicoletti R, Tinelli R, Saliani N, Resta L *et al.* Poor reliability of vaginal and endocervical cultures for evaluating microbiology of endometrial cavity in women with chronic endometritis. *Gynecol Obstet Invest* 2009; 68(2): 108–15.

3. Küçük T, Safali M. "Chromohysteroscopy" for evaluation of endometrium in recurrent in vitro fertilization failure. *J Assist Reprod Genet* 2008; 25(2): 79–82.

4. Adegboyega PA, Pei Y, McLarty J. Relationship between eosinophils and chronic endometritis. *Hum Pathol* 2010; **41**(1): 33–7.

5. Romero R, Espinoza J, Mazor M. Can endometrial infection/inflammation explain implantation failure, spontaneous abortion, and preterm birth after in vitro fertilization? *Fertil Steril* 2004; **82**(4): 799–804.

6. Kamiyama S, Teruya Y, Nohara M, Kanazawa K. Bacterial endotoxin in the endometrium and its clinical significance in reproduction. *Fertil Steril* 2004; **82**: 805.

7. Achilles SL, Amortegui AJ, Wiessenfeld HC. Endometrial plasma cells: do they indicate subclinical pelvic inflammatory disease? *Sex Transm Dis* 2005; **32**: 185–8.

8. Johnston-Macananny EB, Hartnett J, Engmann LL, Nulsen JC, Sanders MM, Benadiva CA. Chronic endometritis is a frequent finding in women with recurrent implantation failure after in vitro fertilization. *Fertil Steril* 2009; **93**(2): 437–41.

9. Kasius JC, Fatemi HM, Bourgain C, Sie-Go DM, Eijkemans RJ, Fauser BC *et al.* The impact of chronic endometritis on reproductive outcome. *Fertil Steril* 2011; **96**(6): 1451–6.

10. Haggerty CL, Ness RB, Amortegui A, Hendrix SL, Hillier SL, Holley RL *et al.* Endometritis does not predict reproductive morbidity after pelvic inflammatory disease. *Am J Obstet Gynecol* 2003; **188**(1): 141–8.

Chapter 44

LH rise on the day of GnRH antagonist commencement

Human M. Fatemi and Biljana Popovic Todorovic

Clinical fertility history

A 27-year-old patient, with a regular menstrual cycle of 28–30 days presented with an 18-month history of primary infertility due to the husband's oligospermia. They had not previously undergone treatment for infertility. The couple had been married for 3 years, but had used oral contraception for the first 18 months.

General medical, family, and social history

The patient had no previous medical or surgical history. She and her husband worked as schoolteachers. Her BMI was 24 kg/m².

Examination findings

A pelvic examination revealed normal external genitalia. A Pap smear obtained without difficulty was normal. Bimanual examination revealed no pelvic tenderness or masses and a normal uterine size.

Fertility investigations

An ultrasound performed on day 3 of the cycle revealed an antral follicle count of 16 (8 on the right and 8 on the left ovary), a normal uterus, and absence of any tubal/uterine abnormalities.

Her serum hormone levels on day 3 of the cycle were as follows: FSH 5.53 mIU/mL (follicular phase normal range 5.2–14.4 mIU/mL); LH 4.36 mIU/mL (follicular phase normal range 1.8–7.6 mIU/mL); prolactin 12.45 ng/mL (normal range 3.20–26.2 ng/mL); and estradiol (E2) 38.03 pg/mL. Her partner's sperm parameters were as follows: concentration: 5 million/mL, motility A+B = 12%, and a normal morphology percentage of 1% according to the strict Krueger criteria.

Diagnosis

The diagnosis of primary infertility due to a male factor was confirmed and the decision was taken to start an IVF/ICSI treatment.

Action plan

In order to avoid ovarian hyperstimulation syndrome (OHSS) due to the relatively high number of antral follicles, the decision was taken to start stimulation in a GnRH antagonist protocol [1]. Severe OHSS is one the most serious, potentially fatal, iatrogenic complications of gonadotropin administration that can and should be avoided [2].

Ovarian stimulation and IVF/ICSI procedures

recFSH was started in the afternoon of day 2 of the cycle at 200 IU/day. The dose of recFSH remained unchanged until day 5 of stimulation. To inhibit premature LH surge, it was planned to administer GnRH antagonist from the morning of day 6 of stimulation.

On day 6 of stimulation (in the morning at 09:00), the patient was seen with a request for ultrasound and endocrine assessment: E2 2630 ng/L, progesterone 1.4 μg/L, and LH 24 IU/L. Ultrasound examination showed the presence of 20 follicles between 10 and 13 mm, two follicles between 14 and 15 mm, and two follicles between 16 and 17 mm. Gonadotropin administration was stopped and immediately 0.25 mg of GnRH antagonist was administered to suppress the LH rise. A blood sample taken on the next day revealed an E2 concentration of 2580 ng/L, an LH concentration of 2.5 IU/L, a progesterone concentration of 1.2 μg/L, and an identical ultrasound picture, but with three dominant follicles of 17–18 mm and a triple-line endometrium of 8 mm. On day 7 of stimulation, 5000 IU of hCG was administered. Fourteen oocytes were retrieved 36 hours later, and one good-quality embryo was transferred on day 5, while seven blastocysts were frozen. Luteal phase supplementation with vaginal administration of 600 mg natural micronized progesterone in three separate doses of 200 mg was applied, starting the day after oocyte retrieval and continued until 7 weeks of gestation.

Outcome

A positive serum hCG 12 days postembryo transfer was detected. The patient did not develop OHSS. An ultrasound at 7 weeks revealed an ongoing pregnancy.

General remarks

This case report confirms the immediate LH suppression after the administration of GnRH antagonist without an apparent negative effect on the achievement of pregnancy. Despite the onset of LH rise, ovulation was prevented, since progesterone levels did not increase. The mild elevation of serum progesterone level (1.4 ng/mL) was not related to LH but to high number of follicles and the E_2 levels [3].

The aim of using GnRH antagonists in IVF is the inhibition of a premature LH rise, which could lead to premature luteinization, follicle maturation arrest, and asynchrony of oocyte maturation.

In all phase 3 comparative trials, in which the daily GnRH antagonist protocol was used, initiation of GnRH antagonist was performed on day 6 of stimulation [4]. However, this choice was not evidence-based and, in principle, GnRH antagonist administration should commence when there is follicular development and/or production of E_2 by the developing follicles, which might give rise to a premature elevation in pituitary LH release by positive feedback mechanisms. Thus the idea of a flexible GnRH antagonist initiation is worth re-evaluating and might lead to a further increase in efficacy.

As published previously [5], fixed day-6 initiation could be recommended in normal responders. However, high responders might benefit from earlier (day 5) initiation of GnRH antagonist. On the other hand, a poor responder could rather benefit from a flexible protocol. Further randomized clinical trials are needed to confirm the individualization of GnRH antagonist initiation.

In conclusion, this case report confirms immediate LH suppression after the administration of a GnRH antagonist without an apparent negative impact on the achievement of pregnancy, despite the initiation of a LH surge, in the absence of serum progesterone rise.

References

1. Papanikolaou EG, Humaidan P, Polyzos N, Kalantaridou S, Kol S, Benadiva C, Tournaye H, Tarlatzis B. New algorithm for OHSS prevention. *Report Biol Endocrinol* 2011; 3(9): 147.

2. Fatemi HM, Blockeel C and Devroey P. Ovarian stimulation: today and tomorrow *Curr Pharm Biotechnol* 2012; 13: 392–7.

3. Kyrou D, Al-Azemi M, Papanikolaou EG *et al.* The relationship of premature progesterone rise with serum estradiol levels and number of follicles in GnRH antagonist/recombinant FSH-stimulated cycles. *Eur J Obstet Gynecol Reprod Biol* 2012; 162: 165–8.

4. Tarlatzis BC, Fauser BC, Kolibianakis EM *et al.* GnRH antagonists in ovarian stimulation for IVF. *Hum Reprod Update* 2006; 12: 333–40.

5. Kolibianakis EM, Venetis CA, Kalogeropoulou L, Papanikolaou E, Tarlatzis BC. Fixed versus flexible gonadotropin-releasing hormone antagonist administration in in vitro fertilization: a randomized controlled trial. *Fertil Steril* 2011; 95: 558–62.

Controlled ovarian stimulation (COS) in a woman with normal ovarian reserve

Shane T. Lipskind and Elizabeth S. Ginsburg

Clinical fertility history

A 33-year-old nulligravida presented with fertility concerns. She and her 35-year-old husband had been trying to conceive with timed intercourse for 2 years. She had regular menstrual cycles and documented ovulation with urinary LH kits on several occasions. Her husband had not fathered any children in other relationships.

General medical, family, and social history

Both individuals were healthy, were nonsmokers, and consumed 1–2 alcoholic beverages on occasion. They reported no sexual dysfunction, and the woman had no history of pelvic pain or infections. There was no history of genetic disorders or mental retardation on either side of the family.

Examination findings

The patient was a well-developed, well-nourished white woman in no distress. Her BMI was 28 kg/m^2. Vital signs were normal and general examination revealed no acne, hirsutism, goiter, proptosis, acanthosis, or abdominal striae. Her pelvic examination was also normal.

Fertility investigations

A hysterosalpingogram showed normal uterine filling and bilateral spillage of contrast from the fallopian tubes. Cycle day 3 serum FSH and estradiol levels were within normal limits (6.2 mIU/mL and 43 pg/mL, respectively). Her AMH level was 3.8 ng/mL. Prolactin and TSH levels were normal. An early follicular ultrasound demonstrated a normal uterus and ovaries, with 8 antral follicles on the left and 10 on the right. The husband's semen analyses revealed abnormal parameters: count <15 million, concentration 10–15 million/mL, motility 15–20%, and fewer than 4% normal forms (by Kruger morphology) on two separate occasions.

Other clinical investigations

Preconception genetic and infectious disease screening were both negative. The husband was referred to a urologist, but further evaluation revealed no underlying cause for his abnormal semen analyses.

Diagnosis

Severe male factor infertility.

Action plan

Treatment by in vitro fertilization (IVF) with intracytoplasmic sperm injection (ICSI) using a long luteal GnRH agonist (GnRHa) protocol was recommended. After documentation of hypothalamic–pituitary–ovarian suppression following GnRHa down-regulation treatment, ovarian stimulation was commenced with 225 IU of recombinant FSH (rFSH) once daily.

Outcome

Despite decreasing and withholding gonadotropins, the patient's estradiol (E2) rose to 5400 pg/mL on stimulation day 11 with 10 follicles per ovary measuring 12–16 mm plus many smaller ones. The E2 finally dropped to 2460 pg/mL on day 16, with large follicles present bilaterally, and final oocyte maturation was triggered with 10 000 IU of hCG. Thirty-one oocytes were retrieved, 18 fertilized, and a single high-quality embryo was transferred on day 3. Nine blastocysts were subsequently cryopreserved. Four days later, the patient presented with nausea, bloating, weight gain, and shortness of breath. Ultrasound examination showed enlarged ovaries and massive ascites. A blood count showed hemoconcentration and leukocytosis (WBC 14 000/μL and hematocrit 52%). A paracentesis removed 2400 mL of ascites. The patient was unable to drink, and required hospital admission for IV fluids, antiemetics, prophylactic anticoagulation, and monitoring.

General remarks

A young woman with excellent ovarian reserve was at risk for excessive response to gonadotropins and ovarian hyperstimulation syndrome (OHSS). Risk factors for OHSS are young age (<33 years old), normal ovarian reserve testing (day-3 FSH <10 mIU/mL, high basal AMH (>3.5 ng/mL), high AFC (>8–12 per ovary), polycystic ovary syndrome (PCOS) (especially with lean body habitus), and prior history of excessive response to controlled ovarian stimulation (COS) [1, 2]. Primary prevention of OHSS requires judicious selection of both starting gonadotropin dose and COS protocol. Secondary preventative measures, such as cycle cancellation, "coasting," cryopreservation of all embryos, and cabergoline and GnRH antagonist treatment remain possible when cycle indicators, such as high serum E2 (>4000 pg/mL), follicle number (>13 over 11 mm in diameter), and oocyte number (>11) are encountered [1, 3].

Studies seeking to define optimal FSH starting doses for presumed normal responders show that doses of 150–225 IU/day usually yield a sufficient number of oocytes for IVF. Moreover, cycle cancellation for poor response is not increased at starting doses as low as 112.5–150 IU, making this a reasonable dose range for potential hyper-responders [4, 5, 6]. There is currently debate surrounding the relative risk of OHSS using different gonadotropin preparations: while HMG and rFSH convey similar risk for OHSS in a general ART population, some have suggested that substitution of LH or hCG for FSH in the late follicular phase for women with polycystic ovaries may improve selection of follicles that are destined to mature while inducing apoptosis of smaller FSH-dependent follicles. In theory, this could lead to an overall decrease in VEGF production by the follicular cohort and lower rates of OHSS. Until further investigation can resolve this issue, however, the decision to use FSH alone or in combination with LH or hCG should be guided on drug availability, cost, and experience [7, 8].

Pretreatment of long GnRHa cycles with oral contraceptive pills for 2–6 weeks may promote ovarian suppression and reduce the likelihood of OHSS. Full-dose (rather than diluted) GnRHa and extended-duration GnRHa treatment may also be used to mitigate ovarian response [9]. Finally, a lower-dose hCG trigger (3300–5000 IU) may be used to reduce follicular stimulation by hCG [1].

GnRH antagonist protocols are a highly appealing alternative to long luteal GnRHa in women at risk for excessive response to gonadotropins. A recently updated Cochrane Review considering 45 randomized control trials involving 7511 patients showed that GnRH antagonist reduced the incidence of OHSS by 60% compared with long agonist protocols and cut the rate of cycle cancellation or coasting in half without any significant difference in live birth rate [10]. Antagonist protocols also enable the use of GnRH triggers, which can virtually eliminate the risk of early OHSS but may be associated with lower live birth rate in fresh autologous cycles (probably due to early luteolysis and luteal phase deficiency) [10, 11]. Pregnancy rates of donor egg-recipients are not compromised by GnRHa triggers, indicating an effect on endometrial receptivity rather than egg/embryo quality [1].

Additional adjuncts deserving consideration are the use of pre-cycle metformin for PCOS patients and dopamine agonist therapy starting with oocyte retrieval [1, 3]. Minimal stimulation IVF or natural cycle IVF with IVM (if needed) result in far lower live birth rates per stimulation than standard GnRH antagonist protocols, which appear to optimize efficacy, flexibility, and safety for most patients with excellent ovarian reserve [12].

References

1. Fiedler K, Ezcurra D. Predicting and preventing ovarian hyperstimulation syndrome (OHSS): the need for individualized not standardized treatment. *Reprod Biol Endocrinol* 2012; **10**: 32.

2. Ocal P, Sahmay S, Cetin M, Irez T, Guralp O, Cepni I. Serum anti-Mullerian hormone and antral follicle count as predictive markers of OHSS in ART cycles. *J Assist Reprod Genet* 2011; **28**(12): 1197–203.

3. Check JH, Slovis B. Choosing the right stimulation protocol for in vitro fertilization-embryo transfer in poor, normal, and hyper-responders. *Clin Exp Obstet Gynecol* 2011; **38**(4): 313–17.

4. La Marca A, Papaleo E, Grisendi V, Argento C, Giulini S, Volpe A. Development of a nomogram based on markers of ovarian reserve for the individualisation of the follicle-stimulating hormone starting dose in in vitro fertilisation cycles. *BJOG* 2012; **119**(10): 1171–9.

5. Olivennes F, Howies CM, Borini A, Germond M, Trew G, Wikland M *et al.* Individualizing FSH dose for assisted reproduction using a novel algorithm: the CONSORT study. *Reprod Biomed Online* 2011; **22**(Suppl 1): S73–82.

6. Sterrenburg MD, Veltman-Verhulst SM, Eijkemans MJ, Hughes EG, Macklon NS, Broekmans FJ *et al.* Clinical outcomes in relation to the daily dose of recombinant follicle-stimulating hormone for ovarian stimulation in in vitro fertilization in presumed normal responders younger than 39 years: a meta-analysis. *Hum Reprod Update* 2011; **17**(2): 184–96.

7. Ashrafi M, Kiani K, Ghasemi A, Rastegar F, Nabavi M. The effect of low dose human chorionic gonadotropin on follicular response and oocyte maturation in PCOS patients undergoing IVF cycles: a randomized clinical trial of efficacy and safety. *Arch Gynecol Obstet* 2011; **284**(6): 1431–8.

8. van Wely M, Kwan I, Burt AL, Thomas J, Vail A, Van der Veen F *et al.* Recombinant versus urinary gonadotrophin for ovarian stimulation in assisted reproductive technology cycles. *Cochrane Database Syst Rev* 2011; (2): CD005354.

9. Damario MA, Barmat L, Liu HC, Davis OK, Rosenwaks Z. Dual suppression with oral contraceptives and gonadotrophin releasing-hormone agonists improves in-vitro fertilization outcome in high responder patients. *Hum Reprod* 1997; **12**(11): 2359–65.

10. Youssef MA, Van der Veen F, Al-Inany HG, Griesinger G, Mochtar MH, Aboulfoutouh I *et al.* Gonadotropin-releasing hormone agonist versus HCG for oocyte triggering in antagonist assisted reproductive technology cycles. *Cochrane Database Syst Rev* 2011; (1): CD008046.

11. Humaidan P, Kol S, Papanikolaou EG. GnRH agonist for triggering of final oocyte maturation: time for a change of practice? *Hum Reprod Update* 2011; **17**(4): 510–24.

12. de Ziegler D, Streuli I, Gayet V, Frydman N, Bajouh O, Chapron C. Retrieving oocytes from small non-stimulated follicles in polycystic ovary syndrome (PCOS): in vitro maturation (IVM) is not indicated in the new GnRH antagonist era. *Fertil Steril* 2012; **98**(2): 290–3.

Errors in dosing medications

Saioa Torrealday and Leo Doherty

Chapter

46

PATIENT 1

Clinical fertility history

The patient was a 37-year-old gravida 0, with endometriosis and diminished ovarian reserve, who presented for evaluation of primary infertility after 6 years of trying unsuccessfully to conceive. She had a significant history of two failed in vitro fertilization (IVF) cycles performed at an outside facility 5 years prior to presentation. She presented to our clinic desiring another IVF cycle.

General medical, family, and social history

The patient had two prior laparotomies for bilateral endometrioma excisions and endometriosis implant ablation. Her last surgery was 5 years prior when she was undergoing infertility treatment. She had not been on suppressive medication or obtained medical treatment for her endometriosis since that time. She reported regular menses every 33 days, lasting 4 days with moderate flow. She did experience dysmenorrhea on the first three days of her menses. She had no other medical conditions and was currently not on any medications. She denied any history of abnormal pap smears or sexually transmitted diseases, and denied any tobacco, alcohol, or illicit drug use.

Her husband was 39 years old with no known medical issues. He was not currently taking any medications and denied any surgical history. He was a nonsmoker and nondrinker and denied any illicit drug use. He had not fathered any children.

Examination findings

The patient was a healthy-appearing woman with a BMI of 20.6 kg/m². Physical examination was remarkable only for her Pfannenstiel incision scar from her previous laparotomies.

Fertility investigations

Her cycle day 3 basal ovarian reserve testing revealed a follicle-stimulating hormone level (FSH) of 11.2 IU/L, luteinizing hormone (LH) of 5.8 IU/L, and estradiol (E2) level of 76 pg/mL. She had an antimüllerian hormone (AMH) of 0.27 ng/mL. Her infectious disease screening for human immunodeficiency virus (HIV), hepatitis, and syphilis was negative. She was rubella and varicella immune and had a normal thyroid-stimulating hormone (TSH) and prolactin level.

A transvaginal ultrasound was performed which revealed a normal anteverted uterus and left ovary. The right ovary had two cysts consistent with endometriomas measuring 2.5 cm × 2.7 cm and 2.0 cm × 1.6 cm. The patient was also noted to have a low antral follicle count (four antral follicles/ovary).

Her partner's serology also was negative for HIV, hepatitis, and syphilis. His semen analysis was significant for a volume of 3 mL, sperm concentration of 58.1 million/mL, 16% total motile sperm, and 50% abnormal sperm morphology (WHO criteria). Repeat semen analysis confirmed these findings.

Other clinical investigations

The patient had had a hysterosalpingogram (HSG) done during her earlier treatment, which indicated right tubal occlusion. She had a sonohysterogram (SHG) done prior to this cycle, which revealed a normal uterine cavity.

Diagnosis

The patient had primary infertility attributable to both female and male factors. The female factors for her infertility included endometriosis, diminished ovarian reserve, and tubal pathology. Additionally, her partner had asthenoteratospermia which further contributed to the couple's infertility.

Action plan

All findings were discussed in detail with the patient and her partner. Realistic expectations were given to the couple regarding the likelihood of conceiving with the constellation of issues affecting treatment. The decision was to proceed with IVF using a mini-dose flare protocol due to her diminished ovarian reserve. Intracytoplasmic sperm injection (ICSI) was recommended secondary to the asthenoteratospermia.

Medication error

On cycle day 2, the patient began her leuprolide acetate and recombinant human FSH (r-hFSH). During the cycle stimulation, the patient inadvertently diluted her leuprolide acetate with progesterone in oil instead of sterile water. This was discovered after 6 days of stimulation when she ran out of her progesterone in oil. At that time she was asked to bring in all her remaining medications, and the error was discovered. The cycle was continued despite the noted error. The patient was reinstructed on the correct method of diluting her leuprolide acetate and for the remainder of the cycle it was administered correctly. All serology findings from her previous monitoring visits showed that the progesterone level was elevated.

Outcome

After 9 days of stimulation, three follicles were greater than 18 mm in average diameter, E2 reached 2230 pg/mL, and she was triggered with human chorionic gonadotropin (hCG). Thirty-six hours later she had five oocytes retrieved; all of which fertilized. Due to the noted medication error, the decision was made to cryopreserve the embryos and withhold performing a transfer during the current cycle. The embryos continued to progress in culture and on day 6 two blastocysts were cryopreserved. The patient returned the following month for a thaw cycle. The two thawed blastocysts were transferred after appropriate endometrial priming with estrogen and progesterone. She remained on progesterone for luteal support after the transfer. Ten days later she returned for her first quantitative β-hCG, which was positive. Her β-hCG was followed until it reached greater than 2500 mIU/mL, at which time a transvaginal ultrasound was done which confirmed an intrauterine pregnancy. The pregnancy was monitored with weekly ultrasounds. Unfortunately, her pregnancy resulted in a missed abortion at 8 weeks. She stopped all her medications at this time and spontaneously passed the products of conception.

PATIENT 2

Clinical fertility history

This patient was a 32-year-old gravida 2, para 1, with unexplained secondary infertility who presented for evaluation after actively trying to conceive for the previous 3 years. She had previously tried both clomiphene citrate and gonadotropin cycles without success. She wished to proceed with an in vitro fertilization cycle.

General medical, family, and social history

The patient had a history of asthma for which she was taking albuterol as needed. She had no other medical or surgical history of note. Six years prior to presentation she had conceived spontaneously and delivered a healthy infant at term. Two years later, she experienced a first-trimester loss requiring medical management with misoprostol. She reported menarche at age 13 years and regular 30-day cycles since that time. She denied any smoking, alcohol, or illicit drug use. There was no significant family history.

The patient's husband was 33 years old with no medical or surgical history. He was the patient's partner for her previous two pregnancies. He was not taking medications. He also denied any tobacco, alcohol, or illicit drug use.

Examination findings

This patient was a healthy-appearing woman with a BMI of 26.3 kg/m². Physical examination was unremarkable. A transvaginal ultrasound revealed an anteverted uterus with normal ovaries bilaterally. A good antral follicle count (AFC > 10) was seen in both ovaries.

Fertility investigations

Her cycle day 3 basal ovarian reserve testing revealed FSH 6.3 IU/L, LH 5.4 IU/L, and E2 level 26 pg/mL. Her AMH level was 3.26 ng/mL. Her TSH and prolactin levels were normal. Her infectious disease screening for HIV, hepatitis, and syphilis was all negative. She had a HSG done prior to presentation, which revealed bilateral fill and spontaneous spill from both fallopian tubes. Her SHG done prior to the planned cycle showed a normal uterine cavity.

Her husband had a semen analysis done which showed a volume of 3.5 mL, concentration of 86.3 million/mL, 53% total motile sperm, and 22% abnormal morphology (WHO criteria). His infectious disease screen was also negative.

Diagnosis

The patient was a 32-year-old G2P1 with unexplained secondary infertility.

Action plan

The plan was to proceed with IVF using a gonadotropin-releasing hormone agonist (GnRHa) long protocol with a daily r-hFSH dose of 150 IU.

Medication error

The patient began her GnRHa on cycle day 21 of her previous cycle. She continued on GnRHa until suppression was confirmed with an estradiol level and ultrasound. At that time, controlled ovarian hyperstimulation was initiated with r-hFSH. On the first day of stimulation, the patient erroneously gave herself a bolus of the r-hFSH. Instead of the planned 150 IU dose of r-hFSH, she administered the entire 1050 IU of the multidose vial. Upon realizing the error, she called the clinic. The provider called the medication manufacturer, who suggested decreasing the dose for the following two days. The patient administered correctly 50 IU of r-hFSH for the next two days, then resumed her regular dose of 150 IU for the remaining days of stimulation.

Outcome

After 10 days of stimulation, 11 follicles were at least 18 mm in average diameter, her estradiol level reached 2490 pg/mL, and she was triggered with hCG. Thirty-six hours after hCG administration, an uncomplicated oocyte retrieval was performed obtaining 19 oocytes. Eighteen oocytes were mature, of which 16 fertilized. Two blastocysts were transferred on day 5. She was started on vaginal progesterone supplementation for luteal support. Ten days later she had a positive β-hCG, which was followed until it reached 2500 mIU/mL. At that point she was followed with weekly ultrasound, which confirmed a normally progressing intrauterine pregnancy. The patient subsequently delivered a healthy female infant at term.

Discussion

In vitro fertilization protocols are complex, and often overwhelming, for patients who present for treatment. The demands of daily injections and the precise timing of the medication administration is an additional stress during this emotionally charged time. Despite pretreatment teaching classes, it is not uncommon to have medication errors occur once the couple return home and are then expected to administer the medications on their own.

In the first case, the decision to cryopreserve the embryos and transfer at a later time was due to concern for oocyte quality and premature luteinization of the endometrium due to the high progesterone exposure. It is known that during controlled ovarian hyperstimulation cycles with GnRHa, serum progesterone levels have been reported to rise in 2–30% of cycles [1]. Some authors have found that elevated progesterone levels may influence the endometrium, adversely affecting implantation and subsequent embryo development due to premature decidualization [2]. This theory is controversial, however, since there are also data reporting no effect on implantation and overall pregnancy rates in cycles with a premature elevated serum progesterone level [3].

One solution to avoid the embryo–endometrium asynchrony that may occur with premature luteinization is to cryopreserve the embryos. The cryopreserved embryos can later be thawed and transferred in a subsequent cycle when the endometrium is more favorable. This method of optimizing the endometrium has shown promising implantation and ongoing pregnancy rates in patients with elevated serum progesterone levels [4]. Additionally, as in our patient, the entire cycle does not have to be cancelled.

In Patient 2, the patient administered more than 7 times her daily dose of r-hFSH. Since r-hFSH is administered subcutaneously, the absorption rate is relatively slow and the medication takes nearly 4–5 days for the steady-state serum levels to be reached [5]. Therefore, the decision was made to decrease the dose for two days prior to resuming her normal dose. The patient's follicles grew at a normal pace and her final estradiol level was appropriate. The patient did well and had a successful outcome from her IVF cycle. Most manufacturers producing hFSH preparations have now implemented pen injectors in order to minimize the risk of similar medication errors.

A provider should be prepared to deal with the numerous medication errors that may be encountered. In this chapter, two relatively uncommon medication errors have been described with the management decisions used to resolve the issues. In both cases, the cycle was salvaged and the retrieval was performed. Both patients subsequently developed blastocysts and became pregnant. Unfortunately, Patient 1 had a missed abortion, which most likely was not attributable to the medication error.

The key to handling medication errors during an IVF cycle is to identify the error as soon as possible and make the appropriate adjustments in order to optimize the chances for a successful cycle. Medical judgment must be used, however, since there may be instances in which the IVF cycle should be cancelled entirely, for example, in cases with a poor response to treatment or out of concern for the patient's safety. However, in most cases every effort should be made to correct the error if this is feasible. In certain instances it may be appropriate to proceed with the transfer as in Patient 2, while in other situations it may be more prudent to cryopreserve the embryo(s) and perform the transfer at a later time when the conditions are optimal.

References

1. Bosch E, Valencia I, Escudero E et al. Premature luteinization during gonadotropin-releasing hormone antagonist cycles and its relationship with in vitro fertilization outcomes. *Fert Steril* 2003; **80**: 1444–8.

2. Melo M, Meseguer M, Garrido N et al. The significance of premature luteinization in an oocyte-donation programme. *Hum Reprod* 2006; **21**: 1503–7.

3. Elnashar A. Progesterone rise on the day of HCG administration (premature luteinization) in IVF: an overdue update. *J Assist Reprod Genet* 2010; **27**: 149–55.

4. Shapiro, B, Daneshmand S, Garner F et al. Embryo cryopreservation rescues cycles with premature luteinization. *Fert Steril* 2010; **93**: 636–40.

5. Gonal-f (follitropin alfa for injections) medication insert. 2011. http://www.emdserono.com/en/therapy/fertility/gonal_f/gonal_f.html (Accessed November 11, 2012.).

Monozygotic triplets after single embryo transfer

Luk Rombauts, Sameer Jatkar, and Mark Teoh

Clinical fertility history

A 35-year-old woman was referred for evaluation of 18 months secondary infertility in the setting of known PCOS and male factor infertility. Her past history included a single-ton IVF-ICSI pregnancy 3 years prior that resulted from her first cycle utilizing a long down-regulation protocol and 150 IU daily recombinant FSH. This pregnancy resulted in a normal vaginal delivery although with a child suffering from Beckwith–Wiedemann syndrome.

The patient again underwent a long down-regulation IVF-ICSI cycle although with 100 IU daily recombinant FSH. Five embryos were obtained in this cycle and she achieved a pregnancy after a fresh day-5 single blastocyst transfer.

General medical, family, and social history

The patient was otherwise well, apart from long-standing polycystic ovary syndrome (PCOS) which was diagnosed after she initially presented with hirsuitism. She had pre-viously undergone treatment with the combined oral contraceptive pill but was men-struating regularly. Her 33-year-old male partner was otherwise well, although past history was significant for a right-sided orchidopexy performed as a child. Family history was unremarkable, although the patient's brother had spontaneously conceived a twin pregnancy.

Both the patient and her partner were storekeepers with no known exposures to envir-onmental factors, regular medications, or drugs. However, the male partner was a smoker of 8 cigarettes per day.

Examination findings

Examination of the patient was largely unremarkable, with a normal BMI, visual fields, and pelvic examination. There was no clinical evidence of hyperandrogenism. The male partner displayed normal secondary sexual characteristics, with both testicles present and of normal volume.

Fertility investigations

Baseline investigations of the female partner were normal except for polycystic ovaries on ultrasound. Blood tests were consistent with PCOS with a mildly raised free androgen index, low normal sex hormone-binding globulin, and day-21 progesterone confirming ovulation.

The male semen analysis demonstrated severe oligozoospermia and pyospermia that persisted on repeated testing and despite doxycycline treatment. The concentration was found to be 0.1×10^6/mL (reference $>15 \times 10^6$/mL) and WBC 3.7×10^6 (reference $< 1.0 \times 10^6$). Anti-sperm antibodies were negative, while FSH, LH, and testosterone were within normal limits. Karyotype was normal 46, XY and no Y chromosome deletions were detected (AZFa/AZFb/AZFc).

Other clinical investigations

Early specialist ultrasound confirmed a viable intrauterine monochorionic triamniotic pregnancy at 8 weeks and 3 days of gestation.

Diagnosis

Viable intrauterine monochorionic–triamniotic triplet pregnancy.

Action plan

The couple were extensively counseled by maternal–fetal medical specialists on a number of occasions regarding management of this pregnancy. The options discussed included continuing with the pregnancy with close monitoring to allow intervention if complications such as triplet-to-triplet transfusion syndrome or selective intrauterine growth restriction were to occur; selective reduction to a singleton pregnancy; and termination of pregnancy.

Outcome

In view of the significant risks of complications involved with continuing the monochorionic triplet pregnancy, the couple elected to attempt a multifetal pregnancy reduction to a singleton pregnancy. For personal reasons, the couple wished for the multifetal pregnancy reduction to take place in the first trimester. The novel approach of an ultrasound-guided monopolar diathermy of the umbilical cords was performed at 11 weeks gestation. The procedure was performed under local anesthesia and was uncomplicated. Although the selective reduction was technically successful, the remaining fetus was found to be nonviable on follow-up scanning.

Discussion

It is recognized that there is an increased rate of monozygotic multiple pregnancy associated with single embryo transfer. This rate is estimated between 2 and 12 times the background rate of 0.4% of all conceptions, regardless of the use of micromanipulation [1].

Monozygotic cleavage may result in shared or separate chorionicity. For monochorionic triamniotic triplets to occur, the single embryo has to divide into a twin gestation between days 4 to 8, with one of the twins undergoing further division prior to the 8th day after fertilization. A number of factors may contribute to this phenomenon. Herniation of the blastomere through defects in the zona pellucida induced by ICSI or artificial hatching may result in mechanical splitting of the blastocyst [2]. Prolonged embryo culture and blastocyst transfer have also been suggested to increase monozygotic cleavage, as indeed is any treatment with gonadotropins.

In addition to the heightened risk of preterm birth, low birth weight, and poor perinatal outcomes of higher-order multiple pregnancies, monochorionicity confers a significantly higher chance of other pregnancy complications. The complications of monochorionicity include feto-fetal transfusion syndrome, anemia-polycythemia sequence, and selective intrauterine growth restriction. Therefore, the management of monochorionic triplet pregnancies requires the input of obstetricians with a special interest in high-risk pregnancy care, such as maternal–fetal medicine specialists, preferably in a tertiary care center.

Early pregnancy counseling with respect to potential complications is an important part of antenatal care. Management options include continuation with the triplet gestation, multifetal pregnancy reduction, and termination of the entire pregnancy due to the significant risk of poor obstetric outcomes or complete loss of the pregnancy. Continuation of the pregnancy necessitates close surveillance to enable early detection of interfetal transfusion and other complications that might be amenable to intrauterine therapy, such as selective laser photocoagulation of placental interfetal vascular anastomoses [3]. Alternatively, multifetal pregnancy reduction to a singleton pregnancy may be attempted to decrease the risk of complications associated with higher-order multiple pregnancies and monochorionicity [4, 5]. Given the monochorionicity, vaso-occlusive measures are required for multifetal pregnancy reduction to prevent acute interfetal transfusion. A number of techniques have been described including radiofrequency ablation, bipolar coagulation of the umbilical cord, laser cord occlusion, monopolar coagulation to the thoraco-abdominal vasculature, and fetoscopic cord ligation [5]. Finally, due to the very high risk of complications, some will elect for termination of pregnancy.

Thus, while elective single embryo transfer is an important measure to reduce the iatrogenic multiple pregnancy rate, patients still need to be counseled with regards to the increased rate of monozygotic splitting (at least 1% incidence) and the potentially high risk nature of these resulting multiple pregnancies.

References

1. Schachter M, Raziel A, Friedler S, Strassburger D, Bern O, Ron-El R. Monozygotic twinning after assisted reproductive techniques: a phenomenon independent of micromanipulation. *Hum Reprod* 2001; **16**(6): 1264–9.

2. Aston K, Peterson C, Carrell D. Monozygotic twinning associated with assisted reproductive technologies: a review. *Reproduction* 2008; **136**(4): 377–86.

3. Chmait R, Kontopoulos E, Bornick P, Maitino T, Quintero R. Triplets with feto-fetal transfusion syndrome treated with laser ablation: the USFetus experience. *J Matern Fetal Neonatal Med* 2010; **23**(5): 361–5.

4. Wimalasundera R. Selective reduction and termination of multiple pregnancies. *Semin Fetal Neonatal Med* 2010; **15**(6): 327–35.

5. De Catte L, Camus M, Foulon W. Monochorionic high-order multiple pregnancies and multifetal pregnancy reduction. *Obstet Gynecol* 2002; **100**(3): 561–6.

Chapter

48

A teenager facing total body irradiation

Kirsten Tryde Schmidt

Clinical fertility history

A 15-year-old girl was diagnosed with acute leukemia. Menarche had occurred at the age of 12 years and she was in full pubertal development at the time of diagnosis. Her periods were regular. She was not yet sexually active at the time of diagnosis.

General medical, family, and social history

A diagnosis of blastic plasmacytoid dendritic cell leukemia had been made with initially only cutaneous manifestations and later also involvement of the bone marrow. The girl had several side effects from the chemotherapy she had received such as polyneuropathy, abdominal pain, and constipation and severe stomatitis. She was living with her parents and had attended the local school up until she became unwell. She had an older brother. In order to ensure the possibility of a lasting cure, treatment with bone marrow transplantation (BMT) was planned. No donors were found within the family, but an unrelated, female donor was identified. The patient was given a protocol consisting of dexamethasone, vincristine, doxorubicin, and asparaginase in addition to intraspinal methotrexate until complete remission. The next stage of treatment was to consist of preconditioning with cyclophosphamide and fractionated total body irradiation (TBI) with a total dose of 12 Gy, and then allogeneic stem cell transplantation.

Examination findings

After remission the hemoglobin was 6.1 mmol/L, leukocytes 3.9×10^9/L, blood platelets 246×10^9/L, and creatinine 34 µmol/L. She was HIV and hepatitis B and C negative.

Fertility investigations

Because she was not yet sexually active a pelvic ultrasound examination was not performed. Neither estradiol, gonadotropins, nor antimüllerian hormone (AMH) were not measured before BMT.

Diagnosis

Imminent iatrogenic premature ovarian insufficiency (POI).

Action plan

Fertility preservation was discussed with the patient and her parents prior to BMT. Due to her high risk of developing POI as a side effect of the preconditioning protocol, and due to the fact that she was not yet sexually active and thus considered unfit to undergo in vitro fertilization (IVF) with oocyte freezing, it was decided to offer the patient cryopreservation of some of her ovarian tissue. Because the initial chemotherapy protocol had not included any alkylating agents, it was assumed that the patient's ovaries would still contain a reasonable number of oocytes. The patient and her parents were thoroughly informed about the procedure by a fertility specialist and agreed to undergo the procedure. As the patient was a minor, written consent was obtained from the parents. Under general anesthesia an entire ovary was removed laparoscopically. The ovary was immediately transferred to the laboratory where the processing of the tissue and the actual freezing took place. The operation was performed in the interval between complete remission and start of the preconditioning protocol. Postoperative recovery was uneventful and the patient started her preconditioning protocol three weeks after the oophorectomy.

Outcome

Histological examination of a small cortical biopsy of the removed ovary revealed primordial follicles. During treatment the patient took the oral contraceptive pill (OCP) in order to minimize the bleeding during menstruations. After the BMT she stopped taking OCP, but her periods never resumed. Levels of gonadotropins were indicative of POI with an FSH of 78 IU/L and an LH of 72 IU/L. AMH was below the detection limit of <3 pmol/L. In order to avoid menopausal symptoms the patient was given hormonal replacement therapy. One year after BMT her AMH was still below the detection limit.

General remarks

Treatment with BMT has a high risk of inducing POI [1]. This is due to the preconditioning protocol, which includes high-dose chemotherapy with alkylating agents +/− TBI. Studies of childhood cancer survivors show that treatment with BMT is an important independent risk factor of POI, especially if the preconditioning protocol consists of TBI [2, 3]. These studies indicate a risk of POI between 66% and 100%. Another important side effect of uterine irradiation is the risk of serious adverse obstetrical outcomes should a pregnancy occur, and this is most likely to be attributable to uterine damage [4, 5]. For sexually nonactive teenagers, cryopreservation of ovarian tissue is the only option for fertility preservation. However, due to the risk of reintroducing malignant cells after autotransplantation of pieces of the cryopreserved tissue, clinicians have so far been very reluctant to transplant ovarian tissue to leukemia survivors. Transplantation of thawed biopsies of cortical tissue from 18 leukemia patients to nude mice caused the development of intraperitoneal leukemic masses in four of the mice [6]. Also, the use of the polymerase chain reaction (PCR) technique has detected potentially malignant cells in cortical biopsies from leukemia patients [7]. However, one study suggests that if the ovarian tissue is harvested and cryopreserved after complete remission has been obtained it may not contain viable malignant cells and may thus be safe to transplant [8]. For teenagers with cryopreserved ovarian tissue the wish to start a family may be years ahead, and the autotransplantation procedure may not be relevant until two decades after the tissue has been cryopreserved. So for these girls other options to make use of the tissue may also be available when the need arises, such as in vitro maturation of the primordial follicles to mature, fertilizable oocytes, or isolation of the primordial follicles with the view to replacing them into the remaining ovary, thus circumventing the autotransplantation. Whether fertility preservation before BMT with TBI is undertaken or not, it is important to discuss the risk of POI with the girl and her parents and the options of fertility preservation available. In a study of young, female cancer survivors, receiving specialized counseling about reproductive loss and pursuing fertility preservation was associated with less regret and greater quality of life [9]. At present however, for many this is not offered.

References

1. Schmidt KT, Larsen EC, Andersen CY et al. Risk of ovarian failure and fertility preserving methods in girls and adolescents with a malignant disease. *BJOG* 2010; **117**: 163–74.

2. Steffens M, Beauloye V, Brichard B et al. Endocrine and metabolic disorders in young adult survivors of childhood acute lymphoblastic leukaemia (ALL) or non-Hodgkin lymphoma (NHL). *Clin Endocrinol* 2008; **69**: 819–27.

3. Jadoul P, Anckaert E, Dewandeleer A et al. Clinical and biological evaluation of ovarian function in women treated by bone marrow transplantation for various indications during childhood or adolescence. *Fertil Steril* 2011; **96**: 126–33.

4. Larsen EC, Schmiegelow K, Rechnitzer C et al. Radiotherapy at a young age reduces uterine volume of childhood cancer survivors. *ACTA Obstet Gynecol Scand* 2004; **83**: 96–102.

5. Signorello LB, Mulvihill JJ, Green DM et al. Stillbirth and neonatal death in relation to radiation exposure before conception: a retrospective cohort study. *Lancet* 2010; **376**: 624–30.

6. Dolmans MM, Marinescu C, Saussoy P et al. Reimplantation of cryopreserved ovarian tissue from patients with acute lymphoblastic leukemia is potentially unsafe. *Blood* 2010; **116**: 2908–14.

7. Rosendahl M, Andersen MT, Ralfkiær E et al. Evidence of residual disease in cryopreserved ovarian cortex from female patients with leukemia. *Fertil Steril* 2010; **94**: 2186–90.

8. Greve T, Clasen-Linde E, Andersen MT et al. Cryopreserved ovarian cortex from patients with leukemia in complete emission contains no apparent viable malignant cells. *Blood* 2012; **120**(22): 4311–16.

9. Letourneau JM, Ebbel EE, Katz PP et al. Pretreatment fertility counseling and fertility preservation improve quality of life in reproductive age women with cancer. *Cancer* 2012; **118**: 1710–17.

A 30-year-old woman with breast cancer

Katrina Rowan

Clinical fertility history

Ms. S. was referred for a fertility consultation 4 days following diagnosis of left-sided breast cancer. The diagnosis was made on fine needle aspiration biopsy following detection of a lump on routine clinical examination. She proceeded to surgical excision and sentinel node biopsy. Histopathology revealed a 16 mm, grade 3, invasive ductal adenocarcinoma. The cancer was estrogen, progestin, and HER2 receptor negative. Given the advanced nature of the cancer, it was deemed highly likely that she would require postoperative chemotherapy.

Ms. S. and her partner had just started trying to conceive their first pregnancy, and having children was a high priority for the couple. Ms. S. had been off the oral contraceptive pill for 4 months prior to presentation. She only had one menstrual period in this time, 7 days before presentation. Both Ms. S. and her partner were otherwise in good health, and had no significant past medical history. Ms. S. had slightly irregular menstrual cycles prior to commencing oral contraception, but no hirsutism, acne, or alopecia. Pap smears had previously been normal but she was due for this to be repeated.

Ms. S. had a maternal grandmother who developed breast cancer in her late sixties, and a paternal aunt with breast cancer around age 40. Neither of these relatives had undergone prior testing for oncogenes. There was no other significant family history, and Ms. S. was an only child. Ms. S. was in a long-term, strong, supportive relationship and was not under any economic strain. Although shocked by the diagnosis, she and her partner were determined to preserve their chances of having a family following her recovery.

Examination findings

Ms. S.'s height was 168 cm and weight 61.0 kg (BMI 21.7 kg/m²). A Pap smear was taken as it was due, and pelvic examination at the time was unremarkable.

Fertility investigations

A transvaginal pelvic ultrasound showed polycystic ovaries, but no other abnormality. Antimüllerian hormone level was high for her age at 29.0 pmol/L. TSH was normal at 1.96 mU/L. Viral serology was unremarkable. A semen analysis for Ms. S.'s partner showed a normal sperm concentration, motility, and morphology.

Diagnosis

Breast cancer in a nulliparous 30-year-old desiring fertility.

Action plan

After discussion of the risks, benefits, and alternatives, it was decided to undertake a cycle of IVF with a view to cryopreservation of embryos for fertility preservation. Given Ms. S.'s young age and the high AMH, it was decided to use an antagonist cycle to minimize the risk of ovarian hyperstimulation syndrome. The initial dose of FSH was 150 units, and the cycle was monitored closely with estradiol levels and transvaginal ultrasonography. After a high serum estradiol (3626 pmol/L) and 24 antral follicles seen on ultrasound on day 5 of stimulation, the dose of FSH was reduced to 100 units daily. After 9 days of stimulation, a trigger of 250 units of recombinant hCG was administered. Although no sperm abnormalities were present, it was decided to perform ICSI on a small proportion of the oocytes as a safeguard against failed fertilization.

Following the end of the cryopreservation cycle, Ms. S. underwent chemotherapy with six cycles of combination chemotherapy (FEC-D). On further histopathological analysis, available after the IVF cycle, slight estrogen receptivity was seen and it was therefore decided for Ms. S. to have at least 2 years of tamoxifen therapy. Ms. S. received genetic counseling regarding the implications of her early diagnosis of breast cancer, and decided to be tested for the oncogenes *BRACA1*, *BRACA2*, and *HNPCC*. This decision was made after the IVF cycle had taken place.

Outcome

Twenty-four oocytes were collected, 19 were fertilized with IVF, and 5 were fertilized with ICSI. At the fertilization check, 16 had shown signs of fertilization. The embryos were grown to blastocyst stage, and 10 blastocysts were deemed of suitable quality for cryopreservation. Ms. S. was physically well through the cycle and did not develop any symptoms of ovarian hyperstimulation syndrome. A second cycle was considered but decided against due to the high number of good-quality blastocysts and the desire to start on chemotherapy.

She was reviewed with regard to her fertility 9 months following cessation of the chemotherapy, and 4 months after commencement of tamoxifen. Ms. S. had not had a menstrual cycle since commencing chemotherapy. An AMH level was measured and this was indicative of a profound drop in ovarian reserve following chemotherapy (AMH <1 nmol/L).

Ms. S. was found to be a carrier of the *BRACA1* mutation. With this knowledge, she decided to undergo a bilateral mastectomy followed by breast reconstruction. Ms. S. and her partner were counseled regarding the possibility of blastocyst biopsy for pre-implantation BRACA testing of the embryos. Ms. S. is to continue tamoxifen treatment up to two years total therapy. At that time, her ovarian reserve and reproductive hormone levels will be reassessed to see whether natural conception is a possibility, but at present it appears likely they will need to rely on their cryopreserved embryos.

Discussion

The first challenge in this case was an estimation of loss of fertility. Reported rates of amenorrhea following chemotherapy for breast cancer vary significantly depending on the type of regime used, the patient's age, and individual patient characteristics [1]. A retrospective review of the incidence of amenorrhea after breast cancer treatment in women age 18–34 showed a 36.9% rate of amenorrhea, but in 83.1% menses resumed spontaneously after treatment, with a median of 3.5 months' time to resumption [2].

AMH has been investigated as a potential marker to help predict postchemotherapy ovarian function, and pretreatment AMH has been shown to correlate with the rate of recovery of AMH after chemotherapy [3], as well as with recovery of ovarian function and bone mineral density [4]. It appeared to be superior to ultrasound antral follicle count and FSH as a marker of postchemotherapy ovarian activity [4]. With a high pretreatment AMH, the possibility of expectant management was discussed with Ms. S. but it was decided, given her strong desire for fertility, that the potential benefits of embryo cryopreservation outweighed the potential harm in her situation. The options of GnRH analog ovarian suppression and ovarian tissue cryopreservation were also discussed, but the evidence of efficacy for either of these treatments was deemed to be too weak for these to be reasonable options for her. Oocyte vitrification was also offered but Ms. S., being in a committed stable relationship, preferred embryo vitrification. An early referral allowing time for ovarian stimulation also facilitated the choice of embryo vitrification in this case.

Ms. S. was warned regarding the theoretical possibility of gonadotropin stimulation increasing her cancer recurrence risk. Early data have been reassuring in that there appears to be no increased risk of breast cancer recurrence following ovarian stimulation [5]. One method that has been employed to reduce this theoretical risk is the addition of aromatase inhibitors [6]. While this technique appears to reduce serum estradiol levels and gonadotropin exposure [6], there is as yet no evidence that recurrence rates are reduced. The use of an aromatase inhibitor was considered in this case but was decided against given the negative estrogen receptor status at the time of IVF, as well as a desire to monitor estradiol levels given her increased risk status for ovarian hyperstimulation syndrome, being young with polycystic ovaries on ultrasound. Another strategy that may be considered to minimize the risk of ovarian hyperstimulation syndrome, particularly in a patient whose embryos are to be cryopreserved, is the use of a GnRH agonist trigger. At the time of this case there was still some doubt as to the efficacy of GnRH agonist triggers, but more recent data have shown that this strategy produces good outcomes with lower estradiol levels and lower risk of ovarian hyperstimulation syndrome [7].

The discovery of BRACA1 mutation in Ms. S. adds extra complexity to the case. Although there is some evidence that BRACA1 mutation status is associated with a poor response to ovarian stimulation [8], this was not a problem for Ms. S. As there is a strong association with ovarian cancer with the BRACA mutation, a future oophorectomy has been discussed, and will be considered most likely after Ms. S. has completed childbearing. The main concern regarding Ms. S.'s BRACA1 diagnosis at present is the potential for passing on this oncogene to her offspring. The couple have received genetic counseling and are deciding whether to test the embryos for BRACA1 carrier status prior to implantation. The embryos were created at a laboratory where blastocyst biopsy is the preferred method of preimplantation genetic diagnosis, and there are several embryos that would be technically suitable for this to be offered. Ms. S. and her partner are still working through the issues that this raises; of particular concern is the incomplete penetrance of BRACA1 mutations and the potential for discarding carrier embryos that may never be affected by disease.

References

1. Hickey M, Peate M, Saunders CM, Friedlander M. Breast cancer in young women and its impact on reproductive function. *Hum Reprod Update* 2009; **15**(3): 323–39.

2. Kil WJ, Ahn SD, Shin SS, Lee S-W, Choi EK, Kim JH *et al.* Treatment-induced menstrual changes in very young. *Breast Cancer Res Treat* 2006; **96**(3): 245–50.

3. Dillon KE, Sammel MD, Prewitt M, Ginsberg JP, Walker D, Mersereau JE *et al.* Pretreatment antimüllerian hormone levels determine rate of posttherapy ovarian reserve recovery: acute changes in ovarian reserve during and after chemotherapy. *Fertil Steril* 2013; **99**(2): 477–83.

4. Anderson RA, Cameron DA. Pretreatment serum anti-mullerian hormone predicts long-term ovarian function and bone mass after chemotherapy for early breast cancer. *J Clin Endocrinol Metab* 2011; **96**(5): 1336–43.

5. Azim AA, Costantini-Ferrando M, Oktay K. Safety of fertility preservation by ovarian stimulation with letrozole and gonadotropins in patients with breast cancer: a prospective controlled study. *J Clin Oncol* 2008; **26**(16): 2630–5.

6. Oktay K, Hourvitz A, Sahin G, Oktem O, Safro B, Cil A *et al.* Letrozole reduces estrogen and gonadotropin exposure in women with breast cancer undergoing ovarian stimulation before chemotherapy. *J Clin Endocrinol Metab* 2006; **91**(10): 3885–90.

7. Humaidan P, Papanikolaou EG, Tarlatzis BC. GnRHa to trigger final oocyte maturation: a time to reconsider. *Hum Reprod* 2009; **24**(10): 2389–94.

8. Oktay K, Kim JY, Barad D, Babayev SN. Association of BRCA1 mutations with occult primary ovarian insufficiency: a possible explanation for the link between infertility and breast/ovarian cancer risks. *J Clin Oncol* 2010; **28**(2): 240–4.

A spontaneous pregnancy in Turner syndrome

Outi Hovatta and Birgit Borgström

Case history

A young girl with Turner syndrome referred to our fertility unit at the age of 12 years by a pediatric endocrinologist participated in a study in which we calculated the numbers of ovarian follicles and related the numbers to the ages of the girls (Borgström *et al.* 2009). She proved to have ovarian follicles in the cortical tissue, as seen in the small tissue piece taken for diagnostic histology. She requested to have most of the biopsied tissue frozen for fertility preservation.

This girl was considered to have a relatively good prognosis for ovarian function because follicles were found. Her karyotype was 45,X, but only 10 metaphases had been analyzed. Such a finding is consistent with mosaic Turner syndrome. She received careful counseling regarding the possibilities of having pregnancies and children. This included a recommendation not to unnecessarily postpone childbearing. She came into spontaneous menarche at the age of 14 years.

The patient later began a relationship with a boy of the same age. These two young individuals decided they wished to have children together, and with the support of their families started trying to conceive spontaneously. She became pregnant at the age of 18 years and was monitored carefully. Ultrasound scan did not reveal any signs of aortic dilatation. Her blood pressure, blood glucose levels, and thyroid function were and remained normal through pregnancy, and she went on to deliver a healthy baby boy with a normal weight at term.

This young family went on to spontaneously conceive another child, a girl, when the patient was 20 years old. Her health remained good, with normal blood pressure and endocrinological health. However, at the age of 22 years, she underwent premature menopause after which she received estrogen-progesterone replacement. Regular health controls were performed once a year. The frozen-stored ovarian tissue was kept in cryostorage in a gas-phase liquid nitrogen tank.

Discussion

The case described here is a very successful one as regards success with spontaneous pregnancies and their outcome. But the situation is often not as good. Risks of infertility, fertility preservation, particular features in infertility treatment, and pregnancy complications specific to Turner syndrome should be discussed with affected couples seeking to conceive and optimal management should be instituted (Saenger *et al.* 2001, Bondy 2007, Hovatta 2012).

Girls with Turner syndrome have normal numbers of primordial follicles in their ovaries up to the middle of the fetal period. Those numbers then start to diminish, but some

26–40% of Turner syndrome women have at least some as teenagers and in early childhood (Hreinsson *et al.* 2002, Borgström *et al.* 2009, Hovatta 2012). Positive signs for having ovarian follicles are mosaic karyotype, spontaneous onset of puberty, and normal serum concentration of follicle-stimulating hormone (FSH) and antimüllerian hormone (AMH) (Borgström *et al.* 2009). Spontaneous pregnancies have been reported among 2–10% of Turner syndrome women (Hovatta 2012) depending on the severity of the syndrome. The incidence of miscarriages in spontaneous pregnancies has been reported to be high (Hovatta 1999), but was also reported to be high in women with Turner syndrome conceiving by oocyte donation (Foudila *et al.* 1999) until it was understood that preconceptional hormonal replacement therapy is necessary to enable the uterus to mature.

Counseling regarding early ovarian failure is extremely important among adolescent Turner syndrome girls, and the possibilities and limitations of fertility preservation should be discussed with them. Ovarian stimulation, retrieval of oocytes, and their cryostorage are feasible among Turner syndrome girls with ovarian function (Hovatta 2012). Cryopreservation of ovarian cortical tissue is possible for prepubertal and nonpubertal girls (Hreinsson *et al* 2002, Borgström *et al.* 2009). Although outcome data remain sparse, the optimal age for fertility preservation in this group is considered to be between 12 and 14 years (Hreinsson *et al.* 2002). In spite of some ovarian function among up to 40% of Turner syndrome women, almost all undergo early menopause, before the age of 40 years (Hovatta 2012).

In case of ovarian failure, excellent pregnancy rates can be achieved using oocyte donation (Foudila *et al.* 1999, Hovatta 2012). In oocyte donation, only one embryo can be transferred at a time due to higher risks of complications in multiple pregnancies.

There are well-known risks in the pregnancies of women with Turner syndrome which should be addressed when a woman with the syndrome is planning a pregnancy. The most severe complication is aortic rupture, which can also occur among nonpregnant Turner women. The risk has to be evaluated before and during pregnancy by measuring the aortic root using MRI, and during pregnancy by echography. The risk is very high among women with bicuspid aortic valves, and the hypertension common among these women further increases the risk. Complications can be avoided by proper follow-up, and by abstaining from pregnancy if the risk of aortic rupture is regarded as high (Bondy *et al.* 2007).

References

Bondy CA. Turner Syndrome Study Group. Care of girls and women with Turner syndrome: a guideline of the Turner Syndrome Study Group. *J Clin Endocrinol Metab* 2007; **92**: 10–25.

Borgström B, Hreinsson J, Rasmussen C, Sheiki M, Fried G, Keros V, Fridström M. Fertility preservation in girls with Turner syndrome – prognostic signs for presence of follicles in ovarian tissue. *J Clin Endocrinol Metab* 2009; **94**; 74–80.

Foudila T, Söderström-Anttila V, Hovatta O. Turner's syndrome and pregnancies after oocyte donation. *Hum Reprod* 1999; **14**: 532–5.

Hovatta O. Pregnancies in Turner's syndrome. *Ann Med* 1999; **31**: 106–10.

Hovatta O. Ovarian function and in vitro fertilization (IVF) in Turner syndrome. *Pediatr Endocrinol Rev* 2012; **9**(Suppl 2): 712–76.

Hreinsson J, Otala M, Fridström M, Lillquist ML, Rasmussen C, Borgström B, Simberg N, Dunkel L, Hovatta O. Follicles in the ovaries of girls with Turner's syndrome. *J Clin Endocrinol Metab* 2002; **87**; 3618–23.

Saenger P, Wikland KA, Conway GS, Davenport M, Gravholt CH, Hintz R, Hovatta O, Hultcranz M, Landin-Wilhelmsen K, Lin A, Lippe B, Pasquino AM, Ranke M, Rosenfield R, Silberbach M. Recommendations for the diagnosis, treatment and management of Turner syndrome. *J Clin Endocrinol Metab* 2001; **86**: 3061–9.

Fertility after conservative surgery for recurrent borderline ovarian tumor

Luk Rombauts, Sameer Jatkar, and Tom Manolitsas

Clinical fertility history

A 31-year-old nulliparous woman was referred for IVF after fertility-sparing surgery for a recurrent high-grade borderline ovarian tumor.

Eighteen months previously an ultrasound for a miscarriage had revealed a left adnexal mass. A left salpingo-oophorectomy was performed along with right ovarian cystectomy and resection of tumor deposits in the left and right ovarian fossae. Histology revealed serous borderline tumor of both ovaries with stromal microinvasion. An elevated CA-125 normalized after surgery. A right salpingo-oophorectomy was declined by the patient in view of her desire for future fertility.

Seventeen months later, a scan following a second miscarriage showed a complex right ovarian mass. A suction curettage was performed and a laparoscopy revealed a 3-cm fungating right ovary tumor as well as deposits in the pelvis. Histology confirmed borderline tumor deposits, without invasion, in the pelvis and right ovary.

Again the patient declined definitive surgery and she was referred for IVF in order to preserve embryos prior to completion of salpingo-oophorectomy.

General medical, family, and social history

The patient was generally well, and her past history was significant only for a cone biopsy performed at the age of 21 years for cervical dysplasia. There was no significant family history of malignancy; she was a nonsmoker; and there was no history of exposure to occupational or environmental toxins.

Examination findings

Examination of the patient was largely unremarkable, with a normal BMI of 22 kg/m². There were no abdominal masses, distension, or ascites noted nor any adnexal masses noted on vaginal examination. There was also no evidence of lymphadenopathy.

Fertility investigations

Hormonal assessment of the female partner revealed a normal mid-luteal progesterone, confirming ovulation and was consistent with her regular menstruation. A baseline transvaginal ultrasound failed to show any recurrence of pelvic disease prior to commencement of IVF. A semen analysis was entirely normal with no anti-sperm antibodies detected.

Diagnosis

Recurrent borderline ovarian tumor.

Action plan

The patient was counseled to undergo embryo freezing in order to defer pregnancy until after removal of the remaining ovary, but elected to have a fresh embryo transfer instead. She achieved a singleton pregnancy on her first cycle with a long down-regulation protocol and a fresh transfer of two cleavage-stage embryos, as was consistent with practice at the time in 2004.

Outcome

The pregnancy was complicated by severe preeclampsia and a liveborn was delivered via emergency cesarean section. The gynecological oncologist attended because of significant intraperitoneal disease including a 10-cm right ovarian mass. A right salpingo-oophorectomy was performed with excision of tumor from numerous deposits within the pelvis. Histology reported high-grade serous tumor with a focus of microinvasion in the right ovary and extensive non-invasive implants in the omentum and at other sites.

She completed six cycles of chemotherapy and subsequently failed to achieve another pregnancy from her three remaining frozen embryos or donor eggs in subsequent cycles.

She has remained disease free in the 5 years of follow-up following chemotherapy.

Discussion

Borderline ovarian tumors (also known as low malignant potential [LMP] tumors) are epithelial ovarian neoplasms of low malignant potential, with histology displaying cellular proliferation and nuclear atypia as in ovarian malignancy but without destructive invasion of the ovarian stroma. Accurate histological diagnosis is essential and formal pathology review should be undertaken by an expert gynecological pathologist.

These tumors have excellent overall prognosis, with a reported 5-year survival of 98% for early-stage disease and 86–92% reported for advanced disease. While borderline tumors account for only 10–20% of ovarian epithelial cancer, they are relatively more frequent in reproductive-age women, with one-third of cases diagnosed in women less than 40 years of age. Thus clinicians are often faced with requests for fertility-sparing surgery.

The management of borderline ovarian tumors can often be complex and should be undertaken in conjunction with a gynecological oncologist. Fertility-preserving surgery can be appropriate but is associated with a higher risk of recurrence than the radical surgery that is still the mainstay of treatment when extra ovarian disease is encountered. Conservative surgery may even be undertaken for those with noninvasive peritoneal implants [1, 2]. This latter group have a very high rate of recurrence, although a second round of fertility-preserving surgery is possible. Surgery for recurrent disease in preserved ovarian tissue is usually curative with no overall impact on survival. Monitoring for recurrence is required after fertility-preserving surgery, with a small potential for progression to invasive carcinoma [3]. Monitoring may be by clinical examination, serial pelvic ultrasound, and CA-125 estimation, the latter being most useful in those with raised CA-125 preoperatively, as in this case [4]. Completion surgery may be recommended after childbearing.

Spontaneous conception may be attempted after conservative surgery, especially for those with early-stage disease. However, in those with advanced disease, as in the case discussed, IVF allows the potential for embryos to be created and frozen, facilitating bilateral salpingo-oophorectomy with preservation of the uterus and pregnancy to be undertaken after curative surgery. This would theoretically have an advantage of earlier treatment, while preservation of the uterus also allows for future pregnancy with donor gametes if desired. However, there is no evidence that IVF worsens the prognosis for conservatively managed borderline tumors or that prognosis is worse if definitive surgery is delayed until after pregnancy is achieved and completed using IVF [5]. Additionally, while there is no evidence that exposure to IVF medications increases the risk of epithelial ovarian cancer, there is some suggestion that those with a history of unexplained infertility may have an increased background risk of ovarian epithelial neoplasms [6].

References

1. Uzan C, Kane A, Rey A, Gouy S, Duvillard, Morice P. Outcomes after conservative treatment of advanced-stage serous borderline tumors of the ovary. *Ann Oncol* 2010; **21**(1): 55–60.

2. Park J, Kim D, Kim J, Kim Y, Nam J. Surgical management of borderline ovarian tumors: the role of fertility-sparing surgery. *Gynecol Oncol* 2009; **113**(1): 75–82.

3. Zanetta G, Rota S, Chiari S, Bonazzi C, Bratina G, Mangioni C. Behavior of borderline tumors with particular interest to persistence, recurrence, and progression to invasive carcinoma: a prospective study. *J Clin Oncol.* 2001; **19**(10): 2658–64.

4. Zanetta G, Rota S, Lissoni A, Meni A, Brancatelli G, Buda A. Ultrasound, physical examination, and CA 125 measurement for the detection of recurrence after conservative surgery for early borderline ovarian tumors. *Gynecol Oncol* 2001; **81**(1): 63–6.

5. Fortin A, Morice P, Thoury A, Camatte S, Dhainaut C, Madelenat P. Impact of infertility drugs after treatment of borderline ovarian tumors: results of a retrospective multicenter study. *Fertil Steril* 2007; **87**(3): 591–6.

6. Venn A, Watson L, Bruinsma F, Giles G, Healy D. Risk of cancer after use of fertility drugs with in-vitro fertilisation. *Lancet.* 1999 Nov 6; **354**(9190):1586–90.

Chapter

52

Successful pregnancy after radical trachelectomy and McDonald cerclage placement in a 42-year-old with invasive cervical adenocarcinoma

Jonathan D. Black and Masoud Azodi

Clinical fertility history

The patient's first pregnancy was an anembryonic pregnancy at age 39 years. She had been attempting to conceive for 2 years. During that pregnancy she was screened with a routine Papanicolou smear that identified cervical intraepithelial neoplasia (CIN) 2 and high-risk human papillomavirus (HPV). She subsequently underwent a colposcopy that revealed adenocarcinoma in situ. A cold knife cone biopsy was then done, which showed FIGO Stage IB1 adenocarcinoma with a depth of invasion of 0.5 cm and positive margins for adenocarcinoma. MRI showed no evidence of parametrial or nodal involvement. For treatment she underwent a robotically assisted laparoscopic radical trachelectomy and lymph node dissection and simultaneous McDonald cerclage placement in anticipation of future pregnancy. The abdominal cerclage was performed using a 0 Tycron suture. The patient was then unable to conceive after having unprotected sex for 24 months.

General medical, family, and social history

Medical history: asthma, polycystic ovary syndrome (PCOS), and anxiety.
Family history: negative for malignancy or infertility.
Social history: the patient had an unremarkable social history. She had never used tobacco, drugs of abuse, or ethanol. She was a court reporter by training and had a very stable home environment and a good support network. She was in a monogamous relationship with her husband. Both she and her husband were of mixed European descent and without any significant familial medical history.

Examination findings

An initial gynecologic presentation revealed a 6-week-sized anteverted uterus with a surgically absent cervix. It also revealed a uterine os, presumably created by the abdominal cerclage that had previously been placed. The cerclage could not be visualized. The vagina was shortened, as is to be expected after a radical trachelectomy. Prepregnancy BMI was 25.53 kg/m² and the remainder of the physical examination was within normal limits.

Fertility investigations

A baseline semen analysis of the husband revealed a volume of 2.7 mL, a concentration of 24.5 $\times 10^6$/mL, and 45% motility. The patient's TSH was 3.59 mIU/L (0.27–4.20 mIU/L) and the prolactin level was noted to be 10.8 ng/mL (4.79–23.3 ng/mL). Baseline follicular-phase estradiol was 15 pg/mL (13–166 pg/mL) and progesterone was 0.2 ng/mL (0.2–1.5 ng/mL). A baseline ultrasound revealed an endometrial thickness of 7.1 mm, a uterus measuring 5.96 cm × 4.98 cm × 5.94 cm, a normal-appearing left ovary measuring 2.85 cm × 1.83 cm, and a normal-appearing right ovary measuring 2.58 cm × 2.50 cm. Hysterosalpingography revealed a normal uterine cavity with smooth contours and patent fallopian tubes bilaterally.

Other clinical investigations

One-hour glucose tolerance test: 138 mg/dL (normal <140 mg/dL [7.8 mmol/L]); PT, PTT, INR were within normal limits. The patient did not have any other significant clinical investigations.

Diagnosis

This is a 42-year-old G2P0010 who underwent a radical trachelectomy at age 39 for invasive cervical cancer, and simultaneous McDonald cerclage placement had been performed for preservation of fertility. Her initial infertility workup was unremarkable except for her advanced maternal age and PCOS.

Action plan

Given the patient's advanced maternal age and small reproductive window, a decision was made to move directly to in vitro fertilization in an effort to maximize the chances of having a successful pregnancy. Additionally, the decision was made to use intracytoplasmic sperm injection (ICSI) as that was thought to provide the highest chance of providing a viable, high-quality embryo.

Outcome

The patient had a successful intrauterine pregnancy after one in vitro fertilization cycle. She underwent ovarian stimulation starting with 5 units of GnRH agonist (Lupron), 225 mg of FSH (Follistim), and 75 mg of hMG (Menopur). The Follistim was titrated to 150 mg and the Menopur remained at 75 mg. On cycle day 12, five mature oocytes were retrieved and fertilized using ICSI. Only three of these embryos were viable. All three were transferred on day 3 after fertilization, at that time they were graded 8AB, 6BC, and 8B. Only one of the embryos implanted successfully. The patient had an uneventful pregnancy until preterm premature rupture of membranes (PPROM) at 30 + 2 weeks gestation. She was administered intramuscular corticosteroids and was given latency antibiotics. She ultimately delivered by primary classical cesarean section at 31 + 3 weeks gestation in the setting of presumed intra-amniotic infection. The infection was diagnosed by persistent *Ureaplasma* growing from two consecutive amniocentesis samples drawn 6 days apart.

General remarks

Conventional treatment for IB1 cervical cancer is a radical hysterectomy with bilateral pelvic and para-aortic lymph node dissection. The patient who desires to preserve fertility poses a specific challenge to gynecological oncologists and reproductive endocrinologists. In a patient desiring to preserve fertility, they can be offered more conservative management in the form of a radical trachelectomy. They must understand, however, that there is a risk of recurrence of disease, infertility, first- and second-trimester pregnancy loss, PPROM, and preterm labor. In an effort to decrease the risk of pregnancy loss, a cerclage should be offered, as it was in this case. Ideally, this would be done at the same time as radical trachelectomy and lymph node dissection. Many patients will require care by a reproductive endocrinologist as patients with radical trachelectomy have been shown to have difficulty conceiving. Factors are thought to include decreased cervical mucos, cervical incompetence, and patient age. In the case of this patient, she had a very small reproductive window remaining and so in an effort to maximize the chances of a successful pregnancy, the decision was made to move directly to IVF without spending additional time on evaluating and treating her infertility. After conception, management by a maternal fetal medicine (MFM) specialist is indicated as patients are at risk of experiencing shortened lower uterine segment, PPROM, preterm labor, and classical cesarean section.

Further reading

Knight LJ, Acheson N, Kay TA, Renninson JN, Shepherd JH, Taylor MJ. Obstetric management following fertility-sparing radical vaginal trachelectomy for cervical cancer. *Journal of Obstetrics and Gynaecology: The Journal of the Institute of Obstetrics and Gynaecology.* 2010; **30**(8): 784–9.

Maneo A, Sideri M, Scambia G, Boveri S, Dell'anna T, Villa M *et al.* Simple conization and lymphadenectomy for the conservative treatment of stage IB1 cervical cancer. An Italian experience. *Gynecologic Oncology* 2011; **123**(3): 557–60.

Petignat P, Stan C, Megevand E, Dargent D. Pregnancy after trachelectomy: a high-risk condition of preterm delivery. Report of a case and review of the literature. *Gynecologic Oncology* 2004; **94**(2): 575–7.

Rasool N, Rose PG. Fertility-preserving surgical procedures for patients with gynecologic malignancies. *Clinical Obstetrics and Gynecology* 2010; **53**(4): 804–14.

Takada S, Ishioka SI, Endo T, Baba T, Morishita M, Akashi Y *et al.* Difficulty in the management of pregnancy after vaginal radical trachelectomy. *International Journal of Clinical Oncology/Japan Society of Clinical Oncology.* 2012.; **18**(6): 1085–90.

Tseng JY, Bastu E, Gungor-Ugurlucan F. Management of precancerous lesions prior to conception and during pregnancy: a narrative review of the literature. *European Journal of Cancer Care.* 2012; **21**(6): 703–11.

Yang KY. Abnormal pap smear and cervical cancer in pregnancy. *Clinical Obstetrics and Gynecology* 2012; **55**(3): 838–48.

Childbearing after conservative management of endometrial cancer

Jen-Ruei Chen and Masoud Azodi

Clinical fertility history

This 30-year-old, gravida 0 woman was diagnosed with primary infertility. She had been married for 1 year without any contraception. In addition, frequent hypermenorrhea and menorrhagia (interval of period 21–25 days, bleeding duration 7–10 days with heavy flow for 4–5 days) were noted. Her basal body temperature revealed a biphasic pattern. Her follicular phase was 10–11 days in duration and the luteal phase was 11–14 days on average. She had not undergone any infertility investigations prior to presenting.

General medical, family, and social history

She was a sexually active, healthy young housewife. Her frequency of intercourse averaged 1–2 times per week, and no dyspareunia was reported. She had never used any contraceptive method previously. She reported having had sexual intercourse only with her husband and was a virgin before marriage. No obvious systemic disease, including diabetes mellitus, hypertension, or thyroid or other endocrine disorder was noted. Her family history was not contributory.

Examination findings

Her body length was 158 cm and body weight was 60 kg (BMI 24.0 kg/m^2). Pelvic examination revealed grossly normal external genitalia, vagina, and cervix. Bimanual examination did not show any tender nodule while palpating her bilateral uterosacral ligament and cul-de-sac. The sizes of the uterus and both adnexae were normal. Rectovaginal examination revealed only a smooth rectovaginal septum. Her breasts were Tanner grade V, and pubic hair was grade IV.

Fertility investigations

Transvaginal ultrasound revealed an antroverted uterus with normal-sized ovaries bilaterally. A 16 mm-thick endometrial stripe was visualized (Figure 53.1). Her estradiol (E2), follicle-stimulating hormone (FSH), luteinizing hormone (LH), prolactin, and thyroid hormone were normal. Her husband's semen analysis was normal (8% morphologically normal based on the criteria of Kruger strict morphology). Hysteroscopy and dilatation and curettage (D&C) were carried out. Unfortunately, the pathology report indicated the presence of an endometrioid adenocarcinoma, architecture grade 1, nuclear grade 1. In addition, there was also strong immunoreactivity for estrogen receptor (ER) and progesterone receptor (PR) in the cancer tissue.

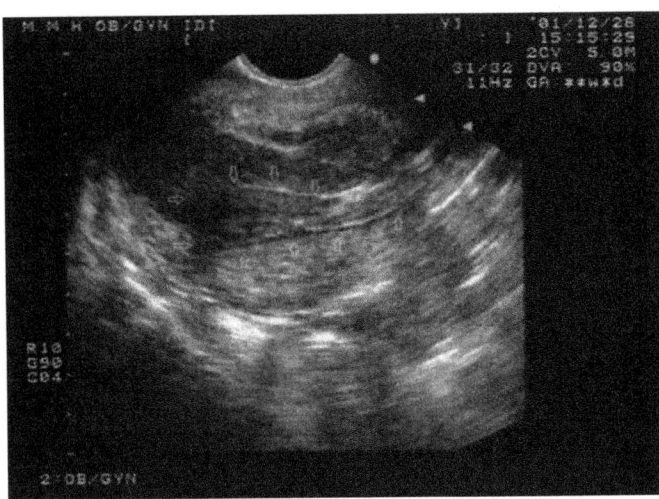

Figure 53.1 Transvaginal ultrasound showed normal uterine contour and a thick endometrial stripe (white arrowheads). Some heterogeneous component can be observed inside the endometrial stripe.

Other clinical investigations

A consultation with a gynecological oncologist was held after the results of the D&C were known. Magnetic resonance imaging (MRI) of the pelvis was arranged for primary evaluation. It showed a sub endometrial zone inside the uterus identical to that seen on ultrasound, normal uterine size, normal bilateral ovaries, and no retroperitoneal lymphadenopathy. Evidence of myometrial or cervical invasion and distant spread of the disease was totally absent.

Diagnosis

Endometrial endometrioid adenocarcinoma, FIGO grade I, clinically confined to the endometrium, and primary infertility.

Action plan

She was interested in preserving her capacity for childbearing. Because of this early cancer with strong immunoreactivity of ER and PR, progestin therapy was introduced. Megastrol acetate (Megace, Bristol-Myers-Squibb Taiwan, Taipei, Taiwan) 160 mg twice daily was prescribed continuously without interruption. Endometrial re-biopsy was arranged at the first, second, and third months after the start of oral medication. She achieved complete remission in one month of follow-up, but Megace was used for 4 months in total.

Outcome

She reached complete remission of her endometrial cancer with Megace. Results of consecutive D&Cs during progestin therapy were all of absence of malignancy or hyperplasia. Megace was stopped one month after the third D&C. Clomifene citrate was then used for her primary infertility. She achieved three pregnancies (one blighted ovum and two term pregnancies). Although there was no evidence of disease recurrence, she insisted on proceeding to hysterectomy after completing childbearing. The removed uterine specimen did not show any residual malignancy.

General remarks

Endometrial cancer is the leading gynecologic cancer in United States and there were 47 130 estimated new cases in 2012 [1]. Sixty-eight percent of endometrial cancer is diagnosed at early stage [1]. It can be classified into hormone-dependent (type 1, endometrioid type, the majority of cases) and independent (type 2, papillary serous or clear cell type, scanty cases) cancers. Surgical staging procedure (hysterectomy, bilateral salpingo-oophorectomy, retroperitoneal lymph node dissection, and/or omentectomy) is the standard primary cancer treatment [2]. Only 5% of cases are younger than 40 years [3] but childbearing becomes impossible after staging surgery in this group.

The pathogenesis of type 1 endometrial cancer is believed to be excessive exposure to estrogen. Endometrial atypical hyperplasia is its precancerous lesion. Conservative hormone therapy with progesterone seems effective in reversing the carcinogenesis of endometrial hyperplasia or well-differentiated cancer. For young females with type 1 (pathological confirmation) and clinical early-stage cancer (disease confined within the endometrium without myometrial or cervical invasion by MRI [4], progestin therapy provides the possibility of cure and childbearing [5]. Megace, medroxyprogesterone acetate (MPA), medroxyprogesterone (Depo Provera), and a levonorgestrel-releasing intrauterine device [6] (Mirena, Bayer Healthcare Pharmaceutical, New Jersey, USA) have been used for this purpose [4].

Several issues regarding the use of progestin therapy in this context merit discussion. First, concomitant ovarian malignancy is occasionally found with early endometrial cancer. Since progestin cannot cure ovarian malignancy, serious adnexal survey with MRI, ultrasound, or laparoscopy before starting progestin is strongly recommended. Second, it is advised to stop hormone therapy only after at least 16 weeks [7] if pregnancy is desired. Continuing progestin is recommended after childbearing if the uterus is not removed. Third, recurrence of endometrial cancer may occur in about half of initial progestin-responders, so D&C for follow-up or hysterectomy is still advised for these cases even without symptoms after completing childbearing.

Dursun *et al.* reported the pregnancy rate in progestin-responders to be 41% [8]. However, assisted reproductive technologies (ART) are usually required in these cases due to their noncancerous underlying infertile conditions, for example, polycystic ovary syndrome and chronic anovulation [5]. When ovarian stimulation is carried out for the initial progestin-responders during ART, the risk of these medications inducing recurrence of the endometrial cancer remains unclear.

Acknowledgment

The assistance of Yuh-Cheng Yang and Hung-Ju Chien in the preparation of this chapter is acknowledged.

References

1. American Cancer Society. *Cancer Facts and Figures 2012*. Atlanta, GA: American Cancer Society; 2012. Available at: http://www.cancer.org/acs/groups/content/@epidemiologysurveilance/documents/document/acspc-031941.pdf. Accessed October 11, 2012.

2. National Comprehensive Cancer Network. *Clinical practical guideline in oncology, uterine cancer, V.1*. Fort Washington, PA: National Comprehensive Cancer Network; 2012. Available at: http://www.nccn.org/professionals/physician_gls/pdf/cervical.pdf. Accessed October 11, 2012.

3. Guidelines for referral to a gynecologic oncologist: rationale and benefits. The Society of Gynecologic Oncologists. *Gynecol Oncol* 2000; **78**(3 Pt 2): S1–13.

4. Sala E, Wakely S, Senior E, Lomas D. MRI of malignant neoplasms of the uterine corpus and cervix. *AJR Am J Roentgenol* 2007; **188**: 1577–87.

5. Kesterson JP, Fanning J. Fertility-sparing treatment of endometrial cancer: options, outcomes and pitfalls. *J Gynecol Oncol* 2012; **23**: 120–4.

6. Kim MK, Yoon BS, Park H, Seong SJ, Chung HH, Kim JW, Kang SB. Conservative treatment with medroxyprogesterone acetate plus levonorgestrel intrauterine system for early-stage endometrial cancer

in young women: pilot study. *Int J Gynecol Cancer* 2011; **21**: 673–7.

7. Ushijima K, Yahata H, Yoshikawa H, Konishi I, Yasugi T, Saito T *et al.* Multicenter phase II study of fertility-sparing treatment with medroxyprogesterone acetate for endometrial carcinoma and atypical hyperplasia in young women. *J Clin Oncol* 2007; **25**: 2798–803.

8. Dursun P, Erkanli S, Güzel AB, Gultekin M, Tarhan NC, Altundag O *et al.* A Turkish Gynecologic Oncology Group study of fertility-sparing treatment for early-stage endometrial cancer. *Int J Gynaecol Obstet* 2012; **119**(3): 270–3.

Fertility preservation in a female of reproductive age with ovarian cancer

Jen-Ruei Chen and Masoud Azodi

Clinical fertility history

A 30-year-old unmarried, nulligravid office worker was found to have abnormal elevation of her serum alpha-fetoprotein (AFP) when it was checked incidentally during a routine examination. The AFP concentration was 103 ng/mL (normal range in nonpregnant women ≤10 ng/mL) initially, but increased rapidly to 1276.9 ng/mL when rechecked one week later. Her menstrual cycle was regular (duration 5–7 days, interval 27–30 days) without dysmenorrhea or menorrhagia. She did not have any symptoms consistent with a high AFP other than recent development of a mild dull pain in the left lower quadrant of her abdomen.

General medical, family, and social history

She was a sexually active, healthy young female at presentation. Her frequency of intercourse averaged 2–3 times per week, and condoms were used for contraception. No obvious systemic disease, bowel habit change, body weight loss, poor appetite, or any self-palpable mass was noted. Her family history was not contributory. Both parents were alive and had no history of malignancy or significant systemic disease. Survey for hepatitis (HBsAg, HBeAg, and HCV antibody titer) was negative. She had traveled abroad during the six months preceding this episode.

Examination findings

Her body length was 170 cm and body weight 50 kg (BMI 17.3 kg/m^2). Pelvic examination revealed grossly normal external genitalia, vagina, and cervix. Bimanual examination revealed a palpable, movable left adnexal mass, about 5 cm in diameter. A smooth contour and mild tenderness during manipulation of the mass were observed. The uterus, right adnexa, and cul-de-sac were normal. Rectovaginal examination located the movable mass anterior to the sigmoid colon. The rectal mucosa was smooth, and inguinal and neck lymph nodes were not palpable. Breast examination was normal.

Further investigations

Transvaginal ultrasound revealed a left adnexal complex mass with both solid and cystic components (Figure 54.1). Its size was 4.51 × 4.33 × 4.01 cm^3. Low-resistance vascular flow was detected in the solid part by Doppler mapping (Figure 54.2). The resistance index (RI) was 0.33 to 0.36 and the pulsatility index (PI) was 0.38 to 0.46. Upper abdominal ultrasound examination revealed no abnormal findings in the liver, pancreas, spleen, or kidneys. Whole abdominal computed tomography (CT) confirmed a left-sided 5-cm pelvic complex

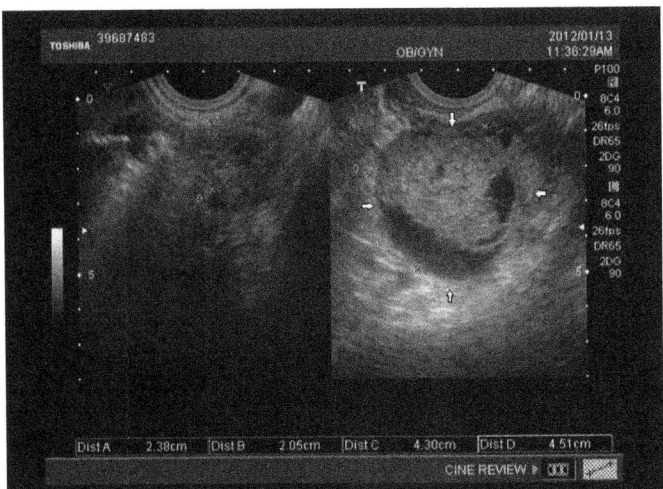

Figure 54.1 Transvaginal ultrasound showed a left adnexal mass with heterogeneous components (arrowheads).

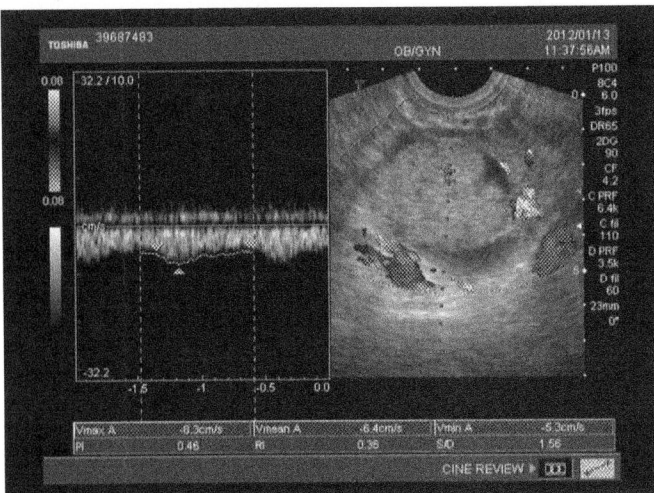

Figure 54.2 Doppler mapping detected low-resistance vascular flow inside the solid part of the tumor.

mass without visible abnormality of other organs or retroperitoneal lymphadenopathy (Figure 54.3). Tumor marker profiling showed CA-125 28.34 U/mL (normal ≤35 U/mL), CEA 2.03 ng/mL (normal ≤5 ng/mL), total beta-human chorionic gonadotropin (β-hCG) 0.6 mIU/mL (in nonpregnant women ≤10 mIU/mL), and lactate dehydrogenase (LDH) 114 IU/L (normal ≤250 IU/L). Routine blood cell count, biochemistry, and urinary analysis were all within normal range.

Other clinical investigations

Exploratory laparotomy was carried out after systemic survey. The uterus, right ovary, bilateral fallopian tubes, and pelvic and abdominal organs were grossly normal. A left ovarian solid mass was found and left salpingo-oophorectomy was done (Figure 54.4). The gross section of this tumor showed an extensive solid part with hemorrhage (Figure 54.5). Frozen

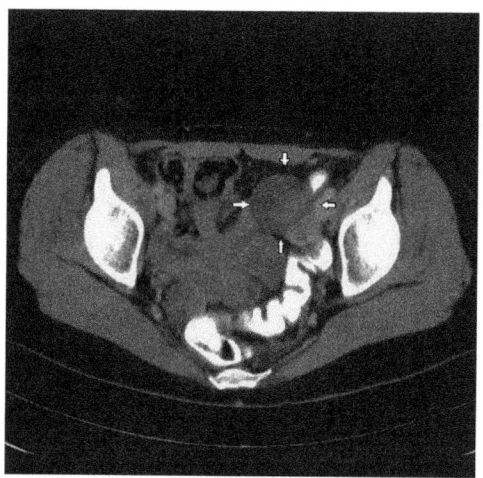

Figure 54.3 Abdominal CT confirmed a complex tumor inside the pelvic cavity (arrowheads).

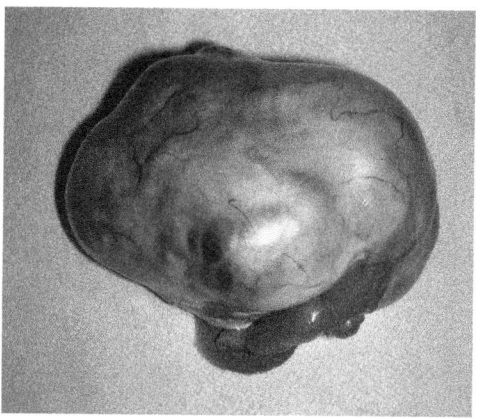

Figure 54.4 Specimen of left salpingo-oophorectomy; the capsule of the ovarian tumor is still intact.

section analysis indicated a malignant germ cell tumor. A conservative staging procedure, including abdominal washing, dissection of the pelvic and para-aortic lymph nodes, and infracolic omentectomy, was completed but the uterus, right ovary, and right fallopian tube were preserved.

Diagnosis

Left ovarian malignant mixed germ cell tumor (endodermal sinus tumor arising from the component of immature teratoma), FIGO stage IA.

Action plan

The patient received three courses of adjuvant chemotherapy with bleomycin (15 mg/m^2 * 3 days), etoposide (VP-16, 100 mg/m^2 * 3 days), and cisplatin (100 mg/m^2 on the first day). The courses were administered 3 weeks apart. Baseline pulmonary function test was normal before starting chemotherapy. Gonadotropin-releasing hormone (GnRH) agonist – leuprorelin 3.75 mg (Leuplin-Depot©, Takeda Pharmaceutical, Japan) – was injected

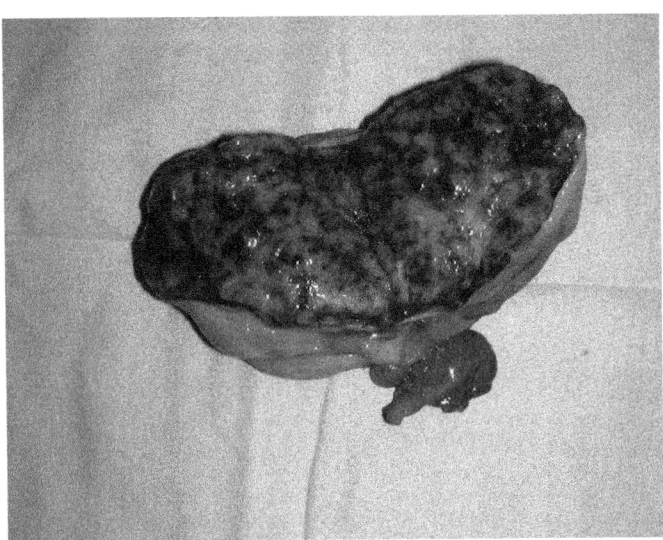

Figure 54.5 Gross section of this ovarian mass showed a solid component with extensive hemorrhage.

intramuscularly every month for three doses. The first dose was given before starting chemotherapy.

Outcome

During the courses of chemotherapy and GnRH agonist injection, she developed temporary amenorrhea and mild postmenopausal symptoms. Her AFP dropped to normal levels (≤10 ng/mL) after her second course of chemotherapy. Two months after completing three cycles of chemotherapy, her menstruation resumed. Recent follow-up (imaging studies and AFP) indicated no evidence of recurrence. She had no difficulty in becoming pregnant one year after completion of her treatment.

General remarks

Ovarian cancer is the second commonest gynecological cancer in the United States. There were an estimated 22 280 new cases in 2012 [1]. The most common ovarian cancers in females of reproductive age are germ cell tumors, followed by epithelial tumors, stromal tumors, and other rare tumors such as lymphoma [2]. Surgical excision or debulking of the tumor (hysterectomy, bilateral salpingo-oophorectomy, retroperitoneal lymph node dissection, omentectomy, and appendectomy) plays the major role in primary treatment of ovarian cancer; however, the issue of fertility sparing becomes another important consideration in young females with desire for child-bearing.

If ovarian malignancy is strongly suspected before surgery, care should be taken to prevent capsule rupture during tumor removal. Peritoneal spillage would upstage the current stage, and the necessity of adjuvant chemotherapy, which is harmful to preserved germ cells, could not be avoided. In clinical stage I epithelial ovarian cancer, and all stages of malignant germ cell ovarian tumor, it is reasonable and acceptable to perform conservative staging procedure without sacrificing the unaffected uterus, contralateral normal ovary, and fallopian tube (fertility-sparing procedure) [3].

Adjuvant chemotherapy with bleomycin, etoposide(VP-16), and cisplatin (BEP regimen) is the standard therapy for ovarian malignant germ cell tumor after staging surgery [4]. Only stage I dysgerminoma and stage IA, IB grade 1 immature teratoma can receive surgery without adjuvant chemotherapy [5]. Fortunately, the BEP regimen has little effect on future fertility [6].

Ovarian suppression with GnRH agonist treatment may reduce the gonadotoxicity from chemotherapy in premenopausal women. In a recent systemic review, subcutaneous or intramuscular injection of GnRH agonist during chemotherapy was associated with a higher potential for resuming spontaneous ovulation and menstruation after chemotherapy. However, a nasal spray regimen of GnRH agonist seems to lack this protective effect [7]. Although the BEP regimen is probably harmless to fertility, there may still be a role for GnRH agonist during chemotherapy to reduce the risk of premature ovarian failure.

Acknowledgment

The assistance of Ya-Ting Jan in the preparation of this chapter is acknowledged.

References

1. American Cancer Society. *Cancer Facts and Figures 2012*. Atlanta, GA: American Cancer Society; 2012. Available at: http://www.cancer.org/acs/groups/content/@epidemiologysurveilance/documents/document/acspc-031941.pdf. Accessed October 11, 2012.

2. You W, Dainty LA, Rose GS, Krivak T, McHale MT, Olsen CH, Elkas JC. Gynecologic malignancies in women aged less than 25 years. *Obstet Gynecol* 2005; **105**: 1405–9.

3. National Comprehensive Cancer Network. *Clinical practical guideline in oncology, uterine cancer, V.1*. Fort Washington, PA: National Comprehensive Cancer Network; 2012. Available at: http://www.nccn.org/professionals/physician_gls/pdf/cervical.pdf. Accessed October 11, 2012.

4. Williams S, Blessing JA, Liao SY, Ball H, Hanjani P. Adjuvant therapy of ovarian germ cell tumors with cisplatin, etoposide, and bleomycin: a trial of the Gynecologic Oncology Group. *J Clin Oncol* 1994; **12**: 701–6.

5. Pectasides D, Pectasides E, Kassanos D. Germ cell tumors of the ovary. *Cancer Treat Rev* 2008; **34**: 427–41.

6. Gershenson DM, Miller AM, Champion VL, Monahan PO, Zhao Q, Cella D, Williams SD; Gynecologic Oncology Group. Reproductive and sexual function after platinum-based chemotherapy in long-term ovarian germ cell tumor survivors: a Gynecologic Oncology Group Study. *J Clin Oncol* 2007; **25**: 2792–7.

7. Chen H, Li J, Cui T, Hu L. Adjuvant gonadotropin-releasing hormone analogues for the prevention of chemotherapy induced premature ovarian failure in premenopausal women. *Cochrane Database Syst Rev* 2011; (11): CD008018.

Mother daughter triplet surrogacy: the first reported case

Joel Bernstein

Clinical fertility history

The surrogate gestational mother (SGM) was a healthy perimenopausal 47-year-old P2 G2 woman. Her biological daughter was a 24-year-old P1 G1 who underwent an emergency total abdominal hysterectomy, conserving her ovaries, for severe postpartum hemorrhage.

The SGM presented with her daughter and put forward the question "Can I be an incubator for my daughter's pregnancy using IVF?", implying gestational surrogacy. This in itself was quite a revolutionary concept coming from a nonmedical person and at a time when the Internet was quite new, libraries were the main source of information and her access to these facilities would have been quite restricted [1].

General medical, family, and social history

The SGM had no significant medical surgical or obstetric history other than irregular menses, probably consistent with her perimenopausal status.

The daughter had no additional or significant medical surgical history, and had no fertility issues with the conception of her first child.

The daughter's husband was a healthy 33-year-old man, the father of their first child. He too had no significant medical or other surgical history.

Examination findings

- *SGM:* Healthy normotensive female.
- *Daughter:* Healthy normotensive female.
- *Daughter's husband:* Healthy normotensive male.

Fertility investigations

   SGM:
- Transabdominal ultrasound of the pelvis revealed a normal uterus, normal pelvis and adnexa.
- Basal FSH 36 and 42 mIU/mL (normal 2–12 mIU/mL).
- Thyroid, prolactin, and adrenal functions were all normal.

   Daughter:
- Basal FSH, 13 mIU/mL (normal 2–12 mIU/mL).
- Thyroid, prolactin, and adrenal functions were all normal.
- Transabdominal ultrasound of the pelvis revealed both ovaries present with follicles.

- Pre-ovum pick-up laparoscopy indicated that both ovaries appeared normal and accessible. (Note that the value transvaginal ultrasound was still being evaluated at that time [2]).

   Daughter's husband: Semen analysis abnormalities:
- Teratozoospermia of 10% (Tygerberg criteria ≥20%).
- Asthenozoospermia of 30% (Tygerberg criteria ≥50%).
- Agglutination 3+.
- Polymorphonuclear leukocytes ++.

Other clinical findings
No factors of note.

Diagnosis
The daughter's surgical sterility could only be treated by surrogacy. The only available and acceptable surrogate that the couple would consider (a gestational surrogate) was her mother.

Action plan
In view of the limitations of assisted reproductive technologies in 1987, the aim was to synchronize the SGM's and the daughter's ovulatory/menstrual cycles by treating both with a combined oral contraceptive pill. Both women had their oral contraceptive pills stopped after approximately 2 months on the same day, and this was assumed to be day 1.

SGM
Induction of ovulation was undertaken with clomiphene citrate 50 mg on days 5–9 of her cycle. An abdominal transvesical ultrasound performed on day 14 showed a 16 mm-diameter single follicle and ovulation was triggered with 5000 IU hCG such that the transfer of the daughter's embryos into the SGM's uterus would occur 48 hours after the SGM's ovulation.

Daughter
Ovarian stimulation was undertaken using 100 mg clomiphene citrate given from days 3 to 7 inclusive of her "cycle". HMG (Pergonal 225 IU) was commenced on days 7–14 inclusive, and monitoring was carried out by transabdominal ultrasound and serum estradiol levels. Final oocyte maturation was triggered with 10 000 IU hCG (Organon), and laparoscopic oocyte retrieval of 11 mature oocytes was performed 34 hours later.

Ten oocytes fertilized and cleaved and five 2-cell embryos were transferred to the SGM.

Serum progesterone estimations were performed on day 2 and day 4 post embryo transfer. Levels of 10.7 and 15 nmol/L were recorded (midluteal range ≥16 nmol/L). In view of the low levels and her perimenopausal status, hCG support (5000 IU) was administered by IM injection every third day.

Outcome
Transabdominal ultrasound examination was performed 33 days after ovum pick-up and this revealed the presence of three regular intrauterine gestational sacs each with a single live fetus. A fourth irregular sac with fetal echoes but no fetal heart was also found.

Three normal live infants, 1 female and 2 males weighing 1.3, 2.3, and 2.3 kg respectively were delivered by cesarean section. The SGM required a dilatation and curettage for retained products of conception 4 days post cesarean section. The children are all alive and well and currently attending university. The SGM, daughter, and husband have also remained well.

General remarks

This case highlights a milestone in the dawn of the assisted reproduction revolution and the many changes brought about by our increased understanding of the reproductive processes and developments in technology, embryology, and medications too many to list. The world's first gestational surrogate pregnancy was described in 1985 [3].

Probably of more interest are the reproductive changes that have developed in the storage, provision, and end use of donor gametes, leading to and being associated with the explosion in commercial surrogacy, cross-border reproduction, and the generation of families for same-sex couples and single women.

This in turn has raised even more questions on a number of ethical and moral issues and has required ongoing reviews of the status of the rights of individuals to reproduce, the rights of offspring generated by these changes, and our rights and duties as medical and scientific professionals.

References

1. Michelow MC, Bernstein J, Jacobson MJ, McLoughlin JL, Rubenstein D *et al.* Mother daughter in vitro fertilization triplet surrogate pregnancy. *Journal of In Vitro Fertilization and Embryo Transfer* 1988; 5(1): 31–4.

2. Feichtinger W, Kemeter P. Laparoscopic or ultrasonically guided follicle aspiration for in vitro fertilization? *Journal of Assisted Reproduction and Genetics* 1984; **1**(4): 244–9.

3. Utian WH, Sheehan L, Goldfarb JM, Kiwi R. Successful pregnancy after in-vitro fertilization-embryo transfer from an infertile woman to a surrogate *New England Journal of Medicine* 1985; **313**(21): 1351–2.

Known sperm donation

Helping siblings in family building

Patricia Baetens and Herman Tournaye

Introduction

Known sperm donation could be defined as a request from a woman to be treated (intrauterine insemination [IUI] or in vitro fertilization [IVF]), using a man's sperm, in order to have a child genetically related to both of them yet without having a partner relationship. From a psychological point of view there are two types of known sperm donation. To define the two types we would use the operational approach: a scale defining the degree in which the procreator is involved in the education of the child. This scale results in a continuum with two extremes: (1) donor versus father and/or (2) known donation versus co-parenthood. To allocate a request for known donation to a particular case, one can use criteria such as: (1) How will the child address the donor? (2) Will the name of the donor be on the birth certificate of the child? (3) Will the donor be involved in important decisions concerning the child such as medical decisions, choice for a school? (4) The extent of contact between the donor and the child and (5) a legal agreement concerning visiting rights.

Two illustrative cases are described below.

Case 1. Intrafamilial sperm donation between brothers

A heterosexual couple from Kazakhstan had lived in Brussels for 2 years for professional reasons. The wife was 38 years old and had severe endometriosis. The husband was 34 years old and had azoospermia. Three testicular biopsies were performed and no sperm were found. They had been married for 12 years. The couple requested an IVF treatment with the sperm of the husband's brother.

Their most important motivation for known donation was fear of anonymity. With the brother there was a genetic link with the child that resulted in a physical resemblance. The genetic health of the family was also an important reason. There was also a cultural aspect involved: the ancestors of the seven last generations of the man should be known. Moreover, there was family pressure in this cultural context: people have an obligation toward their family to procreate. It was a last-chance treatment because of the age of the wife and her severe endometriosis.

The donation would be kept secret from the child, the family, and friends because their cultural and religious norms do not allow sperm donation. They wanted their child to be a normal child, not different from other children within their cultural context.

The sperm donor lived in Kazakhstan and he was married with three children. He spoke only Russian and Kazakhs and psychological counseling, though mandatory for known sperm donors in our center, was therefore, virtually impossible. His wife was not informed. In cases of known gamete donation our center insists that partners of donors are informed and supportive toward the donation, but in this case the couple considered informing the spouse of the donor to be a risk to maintaining secrecy. Informing the spouse of the donor might implicate confusion about parental roles: she might consider this child as the child of her husband. The donation was considered a family business between brothers: there was not even any communication between the recipient wife and her brother-in-law about the donation.

Case 2. Selective anonymous donation

The recipient couple had lived together for 7 years. The spouse was 33 years. The husband was 39 years and had three brothers.

This couple asked for a treatment with the sperm of one of the three brothers of the husband, selected at random. The sperm of the three donor brothers was cryopreserved. At the first insemination cycle, one of the brothers would be randomly chosen to be the donor. At the second insemination cycle a second brother would be randomly chosen, and at the third cycle the brother whose sperm had not yet been used would be the donor. At the fourth cycle the first donor brother would be used again, and so on. The couple and the donors wished to be blinded for the identity of the donor that eventually impregnated the wife.

The most important motivation of the recipient couple was again fear of anonymity. The wife did not want to be pregnant from a stranger. She wanted to know something about the genetic origin of the child without knowing who the actual donor was. Knowing the actual donor would imply a link between the child and the sperm donor. The importance of the genetic link between the child and the husband was the motivating factor, and with the "selective anonymity" procedure the family of the husband would be protected because all brothers were equally involved in this case, with no preferential relationship to any one of the brothers. This procedure protected the couple and their child from potential conflicts with the brothers, as no one knew which brother eventually became the actual donor.

The first donor was 43 years of age. He had been married for 22 years and had three children. He considered the donation as an act of trust: the brothers were very close to each other and it was therefore natural and just to help his brother and sister-in-law. The second donor was 41 year of age. He had been married for 13 years and had two children. He considered the donation as a natural and "technical" act: the child would be genetically related to the family. The third donor was 34 years old and had a girlfriend for one month. The request confronted him, being the only donor without children, with the question whether he, himself, could beget children. He was also very concerned about the health of the future child: he would feel responsible if the child was not healthy.

All the brothers were very willing and eager to help their brother and sister-in-law. Their motivations were slightly different but all three of them agreed that the child should be the child of the recipients; all decisions concerning the child were to be taken by the recipients, the true parents of the child. They respected the privacy of the couple and discussed the donation only with the recipient couple but not among themselves as "donor brothers." The future child would be informed about the selective anonymous procedure.

Discussion

Overview of cases involving known sperm donors

Between 1994 and September 2012, the Center for Reproductive Medicine of the Dutch-speaking University of Brussels received 139 requests for known sperm donation. Of these cases, 39 were requested by single women (28.1%), 65 by lesbian couples (46.8%), and 34 by heterosexual couples (25.2%). In 39.6% of the cases, donors were homosexual men, of whom 18.7% were single and 20.9% had a partner. Another 59% of the donors were heterosexual men, of whom 30.9% were in a partner relationship and 28.1% were single. Finally, 2 donors were bisexual men without a partner. Most of the donors were friends (54.7%). Other donors (50.8%) were acquaintances or were relatively unknown to the recipients, e.g., recruited through the Internet (3.6%). Five donors (3.6%) were partners in relatively unstable partner relationships with the single women who requested the treatment. The remaining 32.4% of the donors were family members.

In 33.1% of our cases ($n = 46$), the request could be defined as a case of "co-parenthood." In these cases the sperm donor will be involved in the education of the child. Single women and lesbian couples opted for this kind of case, referring to the right of the child to have a father (91.3%); the need of a child to develop an emotional, social, and preferential relationship with a man (60.9%); and the right of the child to have access to his or her genetic origin (30.4%). Requests for co-parenthood never involved hetero-sexual couples.

Ninety of our cases (64.7%) could be defined as a known sperm donation; the sperm donor was not intended to be involved in the education of the future child. In the majority of cases (57%), fear of anonymity was the most important reason for requesting treatment with a known donor. Recipients wanted to control the choice of the donor. They were afraid of an unknown genetic origin and wanted a genetic reference for themselves. The right of the child to know his or her genetic origin motivated 45.2% of the recipients. Twelve percent of the recipients preferred a known donor for cultural and/or religious reasons. In 47.3% of the requests, the intended parents were motivated by the wish to have a child genetically related to the partner. The donor was a family member of the partner and therefore ensured the preservation of a genetic relationship with the child.

In three cases the request could be described as a "selective anonymous sperm dona-tion." In these cases, two or more brothers were involved as sperm donors. The actual donor was eventually randomly chosen for each cycle of treatment by the sperm bank. Recipients, donors, and the future child were blinded for this choice and were not informed about the identity of the donor. Nevertheless, the child was genetically related to his social father.

In known donation the most important advantage for the child, namely having access to its genetic reference, is not always respected. In 20.9% (29 cases) of all cases, the recipi-ents wanted to keep the sperm donation secret. This was not the case in requests of lesbian couples and not in cases of co-parenthood. Five single women and 24 heterosexual couples requesting treatment with a known donor wanted to keep the donation secret.

Family donors

Among 139 cases, 45 (32.4%) involved family donors. Table 56.1 summarizes the relation-ship with the recipients. Only one family donor was involved as a co-parent in a request by a lesbian couple. All other family donors were involved in known donation, without any responsibility of the donor toward the education of the future child. In cases of known dona-tion with a family donor, one request came from a single woman having oocyte donation as well, 12 requests came from lesbian couples, and 31 came from heterosexual couples. In fam-ily donor requests, 73.4% were sibling donations, of which 46.7% were brother-to-brother donation ($n = 21$). Three cases were "selective anonymous sperm donation."

Table 56.1 Types of family donor

Relationship of donor	Number (percentage of total)
Brother of the male partner	18 (40%)
Two or more brothers of the male partner	3 (6.7%)
Brother of the female partner	8 (17.8%)
Father of the male partner	9 (20%)
Father of the female partner	1 (2.2%)
Brother-in-law	1 (2.2%)
Brother of the single mother + oocyte donation	1 (2.2%)
Brother of the biological mother + oocyte donation of the social mother	3 (6.7%)
Nephew of the social mother	1 (2.2%)
	45 (100%)

In 23 cases involving a family donor, the recipients wished to keep the donation secret: 13 cases of donation with a brother of the male partner ($n = 21$) and 8 cases of intergenerational donation, i.e., father-to-son donation ($n = 9$).

Conclusion

Known sperm donation involves the use of sperm from a man known to the recipient or recipient couple. Almost one third of known donations involved a family donor ($n = 45$) of whom the majority (46.7%) were brother-to-brother donations ($n = 21$). In these sibling donations, the majority of the intended parents ($n = 13$) wanted to keep the treatment secret. Heterosexual couples tend to withhold this information from the child because of fear of confusion about parental roles. They choose a family donor in order to preserve a genetic relationship with the partner but at the cost of withholding genetic information from the child.

The potential for conflict is higher in known donation than in anonymous donation. Our center therefore claims the right to refuse a request for known sperm donation if the situation involves too many factors that might endanger the welfare of the child. Sixty-seven percent of the requests were accepted for treatment, 21.6% of the recipients chose another alternative before eventually starting their treatment, and 11.4% became pregnant without our intervention. Sixty percent of requests with family donors were accepted, of which 16 involved a brother and 28.9% of the recipients chose another alternative of which 5 involved a brother including one selective anonymous sperm donation.

A 5-year-old with pelvic rhabdomyosarcoma

Alison Fernbach and Jennifer Levine

Clinical fertility history

D.I. was a 5-year-old girl who presented with a several-week history of constipation, pain with urination, increasing abdominal girth, and occasional pain in her left leg. She was seen by her pediatrician, who palpated an abdominal/pelvic mass. An abdominal sonogram showed a 6–7 cm pelvic mass, arising from the apex of the vagina, displacing the uterus and ovaries anteriorly and the rectum posteriorly. She also had hydronephrosis of the left kidney and mild hydronephrosis of the right kidney. A biopsy of the mass was consistent with embryonal rhabdomyosarcoma. Metastatic workup was negative.

Her treatment plan, according to a Children's Oncology Group protocol, consisted of 14 cycles of vincristine, actinomycin, and cyclophosphamide (with a planned cumulative dose of 16.8 g/m^2) and 3600 cGy of radiation to the pelvis in 20 fractions.

General medical, family, and social history

D.I. was born at full term via normal spontaneous vaginal delivery, and weighed 3.6 kg. She had been well prior to her current diagnosis. She had no known drug allergies and lived at home with her parents. Her father was 32 years old and healthy. Her mother was 28 years old with no medical issues. She had an older sister and two younger brothers, all of whom were healthy. D.I. had reached all developmental milestones and was in kindergarten. Her mother worked as a principal for a middle school and her father was a rabbi at the local orthodox synagogue.

Examination findings

An evaluation by the medical team revealed a well-nourished, well-developed, 5-year-old girl with abdominal distension and a large palpable abdominal mass. She was premenarchal with unremarkable Tanner stage 1 breast and pubic hair development.

Fertility investigations

As the patient was pre-pubertal, no additional fertility investigations were relevant at the time. However, the imaging that was part of D.I.'s disease evaluation noted an age-appropriate presence of uterus, with the ovaries not visualized. The mass did not involve the uterus or ovaries.

Diagnosis

D.I. was at risk for chemotherapy- and radiation therapy-induced gonadal dysfunction, including delayed or arrested puberty, premature menopause, and infertility.

Action plan

There were two options available at the time for this prepubertal patient to prevent or diminish gonadal dysfunction and protect her fertility. These included ovarian transposition (oophoropexy) and ovarian tissue cryopreservation. Ovarian transposition involves laparoscopically relocating the ovaries away from the field of radiation. Reports of the efficacy of this modality in preserving ovarian function range from 50% to 90% [1]. With ovarian tissue cryopreservation, ovarian tissue is removed at the time of diagnosis and cryopreserved and stored for future use.

Currently, ovarian tissue cryopreservation is experimental and no pregnancies have occurred utilizing the reimplantation of ovarian tissue harvested before puberty [2]. However, this is the only option for cryopreservation available to prepubertal females. Both procedures can be performed at the time of biopsy or resection of the mass or at the time of central venous catheter placement to minimize anesthesia risks. Both options were discussed thoroughly with both parents, who ultimately decided on both procedures. The family was able to secure resources to pay the US$12 000 for the ovarian tissue retrieval and cryopreservation [3].

Outcome

The patient completed therapy with minimal complications. At age 10 years the patient remained Tanner I and had not yet begun to menstruate. Hormone levels determined at this time to evaluate ovarian reserve showed the following:

- FSH 58.8 mIU/mL (prepubertal <5.0 mIU/mL; postpubertal: <15 mIU/mL; postmenopausal >20 mIU/mL).
- LH 19 mIU/mL (prepubertal <2.0 mIU/mL; postpubertal <15.0 mIU/mL; postmenopausal >20.0 mIU/mL).

On the basis of these values, she was referred to a pediatric endocrinologist, who ordered more tests and ultimately diagnosed her with arrested puberty and ovarian failure. Patient D.I. required hormone replacement therapy to initiate puberty. The ovarian tissue remains cryopreserved.

General remarks

Because of the patient's age and her prepubertal status, her options for fertility preservation were limited. Even though this child had her ovaries transposed out of the field of radiation, the exposure to high doses of cyclophosphamide and the scatter associated with radiation likely contributed to an accelerated decline in follicle number, resulting in ovarian failure and early menopause.

In contrast to embryo or oocyte cryopreservation, ovarian tissue cryopreservation is a fertility preservation option available to all premenopausal females that does not require any delay in therapy. Thawed ovarian tissue can be re-transplanted either orthotopically into the adnexal space or heterotopically into forearm or underarm skin or in the abdominal wall. In this method, physiological conditions are at least temporarily restored, and a spontaneous pregnancy may be possible or pregnancy may be achieved through assisted reproduction. This option has been successfully performed but has achieved pregnancies in only a limited number of adult women, with 10 pregnancies reported [4]. While it appears that cryopreserved ovarian tissue can survive years of freezing, once it is transplanted the life-span of ovarian tissue is limited [4]. In some cases there is the potential risk of re-implanting tissue that may be contaminated with cancer cells [4]. Research is ongoing to develop methods of in vitro maturation of oocytes [5].

Ethnic and cultural mores often influence the decisions that parents make about preserving the reproductive potential of their children when faced with the possibility of infertility. According to the Jewish religion, the obligations "to be fruitful and multiply" and "to preserve the sanctity of marriage" play a crucial role in the decision whether certain forms of reproductive technologies are permitted [6]. The obligation "to be fruitful and multiply" allows for assisted reproductive technology when it is medically indicated for a couple to have children. Although donor gametes are not allowed because that would break the sacred marital bond between a couple, ovarian tissue transplantation is not objectionable if the tissue is being transplanted back into the same woman. Ovary tissue donation may also be permitted if the egg is being ovulated in the body of the intended mother and the sanctity of marriage is preserved [6].

In this case, ovarian tissue cryopreservation would therefore be permitted for this patient. Although the method is still experimental, this research is acceptable because it potentially could promote life and allow this child to fulfill the obligation of being fruitful in the future [6].

References

1. Wo JY, Vaswanathan AN. Impact of radiotherapy on fertility, pregnancy, and neonatal outcomes in female cancer patients. *Int J Radiat Oncol Biol Phys* 2009; 73: 1304–12.

2. Gracia C, Chang J, Kondapalli L *et al.* Ovarian tissue cryopreservation for fertility preservation in cancer patients: Successful establishment and feasibility of a multidisciplinary collaboration. *J Assist Reprod Genet* 2012; 29: 495–502.

3. Livestrong Foundation. Parenthood Options for Women. Ovarian Tissue Freezing. Austin, TX: Livestrong Foundation; 2012. http://www.fertilehope.

org/learn-more/cancer-and-fertility-info/parenthood-options-women.cfm#TID6. Accessed October 20, 2012.

4. Lawrenz B, Rothmund R, Neunhoeffer E *et al.* Fertility preservation in prepubertal girls prior to chemotherapy and radiotherapy – review of the literature. *J Pediatr Adolesc Gynecol* 2012; 25: 284–8.

5. Ginsberg JP. New advances in fertility preservation for pediatric cancer patients. *Curr Opin Pediatr* 2011; 23: 9–13.

6. Silber SJ. Judaism and reproductive technology. *Cancer Treat Res* 2010; 156: 471–80.

Co-fatherhood

Same-sex male couple and IVF

Saioa Torrealday and Dorothy A. Greenfeld

Clinical fertility history

L.S. and M.D. presented to the IVF Center to discuss fertility options considering their same-sex relationship. Mr. S. and Mr. D. reported that they had been in a committed, monogamous relationship for the previous 8 years. They had adopted two sons together who were 15 and 17 years of age, respectively. The couple was interested in having a baby using a gestational surrogate and an egg donor.

General medical, family, and social history

L.S. was a 37-year-old Hispanic man who had no known medical issues. He was not taking any medication and denied any surgical history. L.S. was a nonsmoker and nondrinker and denied any illicit drug use. He had not fathered any children in previous relationships.

M.D. was a 39-year-old Hispanic man with a history of asthma. He required an albuterol inhaler only on an as-needed basis. He had had two prior knee surgeries and an appendectomy. M.D. was a nonsmoker and a social drinker. He denied any illicit drug use. He reported that he had not fathered any children in previous relationships.

Examination findings

L.S. was a healthy-appearing male with a BMI of 18.7 kg/m^2. Physical examination was unremarkable. Similarly, M.D. was a healthy-appearing male with a BMI of 20.2 kg/m^2. M.D.'s physical examination was only remarkable for his appendectomy and knee incisional scars.

Fertility investigations

Both L.S. and M.D. underwent a full infectious disease screen to include human immunodeficiency virus (HIV), hepatitis, cytomegalovirus (CMV), human T-lymphotropic virus (HTLV), gonorrhea, chlamydia, and syphilis.

L.S. had a normal semen analysis that revealed a volume of 3.0 mL, sperm concentration of 81.5 million/mL, 61% total motile sperm, and 30% abnormal sperm morphology.

M.D.'s semen analysis showed slight asthenospermia. The semen analysis was significant for a volume of 3.5 mL, sperm concentration of 39.3 million/mL, 31% total motile sperm, and 35% abnormal sperm morphology.

Anonymous donor

The couple elected to use an anonymous egg donor selected through the Fertility Center donor database. The anonymous donor (A.D.) was medically and psychologically screened prior to acceptance into the donor program.

A.D. was a 25-year-old gravida 2, para 2 with no known medical conditions or previous surgeries. She was not taking any medication and had had two uncomplicated, term vaginal deliveries. She was a nonsmoker and nondrinker and denied any illicit drug use. Her motivation to become an egg donor stemmed from a close family member being unable to bear children. She was currently married with two healthy children.

A.D.'s cycle day 3 basal ovarian reserve testing revealed a follicle-stimulating hormone (FSH) level of 7.2 IU/L, luteinizing hormone (LH) of 5.8 IU/L, and estradiol (E2) of 24 pg/mL. She had an antimüllerian hormone (AMH) level of 2.27 ng/mL. Her infectious disease screening for human immunodeficiency virus (HIV), hepatitis, and syphilis was negative. Her gonorrhea and chlamydia cultures were also negative. She had a normal thyroid-stimulating hormone (TSH) and prolactin level. A transvaginal ultrasound was performed which revealed an anteverted uterus and normal bilateral adnexa. Her antral follicle count was >10 per ovary.

Gestational carrier

L.S.'s sister-in-law, J.C., offered to be the gestational carrier for the couple. J.C. underwent both medical and psychological evaluation prior to participation. Although she was eager to help carry the baby for L.S. and M.D., she was clear that she did not want to be genetically related to the baby.

J.C. was a 31-year-old gravida 4, para 3 with no known medical issues. She took only a daily vitamin. She reported three spontaneous vaginal deliveries at term after uncomplicated pregnancies. She had had one spontaneous first-trimester loss in the previous year which did not require medical or surgical management. A nonsmoker and nondrinker, she also denied any illicit drug use. She was currently married with three children aged 2, 5, and 7 years.

J.C. had an infectious disease screen performed, which was negative. Her serum drug toxicology screen was also negative. Her prolactin and TSH levels were within normal limits. A sonohystogram was performed, which showed a normal uterine cavity.

Diagnosis

The couple had primary infertility due to the nature of their same-sex relationship.

Action plan

After thorough discussion with L.S. and M.D. they wished to proceed with an IVF cycle using the anonymous egg donor selected (A.D.) with J.C. as the gestational carrier. Since both L.S. and M.D. wished to be genetically related to the offspring, the decision was made to fertilize half the oocytes with sperm from L.S. and half with the sperm from M.D. They both clearly understood that the offspring would be genetically related to only one of them.

A.D. started her IVF cycle using the long agonist protocol. J.C.'s recipient cycle, which consisted of ovarian suppression and priming of the uterus in anticipation for the transfer, was synchronized with A.D.'s IVF cycle.

Outcome

After 10 days of stimulation, nine follicles were greater than 18 mm in average diameter, E2 reached 3530 pg/mL, and A.D. was triggered with human choriogonadotropin (hCG). Thirty-six hours later A.D. had 18 oocytes retrieved. Half of the oocytes were fertilized with

L.S.'s sperm and the other half with M.D.'s sperm. The embryos continued to progress in culture and on day 5 two blastocysts were transferred into J.C.'s primed uterus. The decision was made to transfer the two best-quality embryos regardless of the sperm origin. The two blastocysts happened to be one from each of the partners. The couple did not wish to know from which cohort the embryos were derived. Following the transfer, J.C. remained on vaginal progesterone for luteal phase support. Ten days later, J.C. had her first quantitative β-hCG which was 255 mIU/ml. Her β-hCG was followed until it reached greater than 2500 mIU/mL, at which time an ultrasound was done. A dichorionic-diamniotic twin pregnancy was diagnosed on her first ultrasound. Weekly ultrasounds were performed until 10 weeks gestation at which time the progesterone was discontinued. The twin pregnancy continued to progress without complications until term. At 38 weeks gestation, J.C. delivered a healthy boy and a healthy girl via cesarean section.

Discussion

The ongoing gay civil rights movement has encouraged gay men and women to be open about their homosexuality, open about their relationships, and open about choosing to have children within the context of those relationships. As a result, gay couples increasingly seek parenthood through assisted reproductive technology (ART). For gay men the treatment involves IVF with a gestational surrogate, an egg donor, and the sperm of one (or both) of the male partners.

In most cases, the couple is very clear about which one will provide the sperm. It may be that he is older, or has "better genes," or is more concerned about having a biological connection to the offspring. Typically the couple has given this a great deal of thought and made the decision before proceeding to treatment. In this particular case, the couple had equal interest in a biological connection to the offspring and requested having half of the oocytes inseminated with one partner's sperm and half with the other partner's sperm, hoping to transfer a good-quality embryo from each. They were counseled at the onset about the possibility of treatment failure or of having only one embryo successfully implant.

This couple (L.S. and M.D.) had been in a committed relationship for 8 years. They have two adopted children. When a baby they had been foster-parenting was returned to his biological mother, and after L.S.'s sympathetic sister-in-law offered to carry a pregnancy for them, they sought reproductive assistance from our program. The gestational surrogate was a 31-year-old woman who had successfully given birth to two children. The couple was matched to an anonymous oocyte donor who was 25 years old, married, and the mother of two children. Both the gestational surrogate and the oocyte donor met medical and psychological criteria for acceptance in our program. The transfer of an embryo from each father was successful and the gestational surrogate gave birth to a boy and a girl (twins who are in fact half-siblings).

Programs offering fertility services routinely treat lesbians but have been more resistant to accepting gay men for treatment. Entrenched stereotypes about gay fathers – that their children will be stigmatized and are more likely to be gay – has led to this resistance. Several studies have looked at the social and psychological well-being of children and adolescents raised in same-sex households and determined that in terms of personality development, psychological development, and gender identity they are not more likely to become gay and are not measurably different from children raised in heterosexual households.

Providers offering IVF to gay male couples need to be respectful of same-sex relationships and to demonstrate an appreciation of the challenges unique to gay men seeking fatherhood together.

Further reading

Bergman K, Rubio RJ, Green RJ, Padron E. Gay men who become fathers via surrogacy: the transition to parenthood. *J GLBT Fam Stud* 2010; **6**: 111–41.

Ethics Committee of the American Society for Reproductive Medicine. Access to fertility treatment by gays, lesbians, and unmarried persons. *Fertil Steril* 2006; **86**: 1333–5.

Greenfeld DA, Seli E. Gay men choosing parenthood through assisted reproduction: medical and psychological considerations. *Fertil Steril* 2011; **95**: 225–9.

MacCallam F, Lycett E, Murray C *et al.* Surrogacy: the experience of commissioning couples. *Hum Reprod* 2003; **18**: 1334–42.

Tasker F. Lesbian mothers, gay fathers and their children: A review. *J Dev Behav Pediatr* 2005; **26**: 224–40.

Chapter

59

Sensorineural hearing loss following ovarian stimulation

Bala Karunakaran, Nicholas Brook, Daniel Hajioff, Geoffrey Trew, and Theo Joseph

Clinical fertility history

A 28-year-old woman diagnosed with primary infertility secondary to tubal pathology presented for IVF treatment. She had 16 mg of buserelin over 23 days to achieve ovarian suppression, followed by a daily combination of 150 IU of Puregon (follitropin beta) and 500 µg buserelin. The patient presented on day 9 of gonadotropin stimulation, reporting acute-onset left-sided hearing loss, tinnitus, and rotational vertigo. She did not report any symptoms of ovarian hyperstimulation, such as vomiting, diarrhea, weight gain, abdominal bloating, or distension.

General medical, family, and social history

This patient did not have any previous hearing problems. She did not have any past medical history and was a nonsmoker.

Fertility investigation

Her estrogen level was normal and her liver function tests were normal. Previous fertility investigations were all normal apart from revealing tubal pathology.

Examination finding

The patient was examined one day following onset of symptoms. The otological examination revealed normal tympanic membranes and positive Rinne tests with a Weber test lateralizing to the right. A full neurological examination, including cranial nerve examination, was otherwise unremarkable. General systemic examination was also unremarkable.

Pure-tone audiometry was found to be within normal values on the right but no measurable hearing at the left. An MRI scan showed normal internal acoustic meati and posterior cranial fossa.

Her biochemistry findings including full blood count, erythrocyte sedimentation rate, sodium, potassium, creatinine, calcium, random glucose, total cholesterol, triglycerides, thyroid-stimulating hormone, free tetraiodothyronine, immunoglobulins A, G, and M, bilirubin, albumin, alkaline phosphatase, aspartate and alanine transaminases, and anti-neutrophil cytoplasm antibody were all within the normal range.

Diagnosis and action plan

A diagnosis of sensorineural hearing loss was made.

Course of treatment

The patient was treated with corticosteroids (hydrocortisone 100 mg four times a day), and aciclovir (200 mg PO five times a day) for 5 days. Follow-up audiology, 3 days later, showed improved air conduction but still no detectable hearing in the left ear. The vertigo had subsided. At the 6-week follow-up appointment the findings were identical. At 8 months, some mild improvement was noted at pure-tone audiometry, but the overall pattern of hearing was not significantly changed.

General remarks

Sudden sensorineural hearing loss presents rarely, with an annual incidence of 5–20 per 100 000 [1]. Presentation of sensorineural deafness following gonadotropin stimulation is therefore a rare phenomenon. Thus it will be impossible to record a sufficient case series to establish the link between sudden sensorineural hearing loss and gonadotropin stimulation.

Hanna described cases of unilateral hearing loss in women using the combined oral contraceptive pill [2]. Hanna postulated that this hearing loss could be secondary to a thrombotic event, which is a known risk factor of the combined oral contraceptive pill. As the middle ear features the terminal branch of the posterior cerebral artery, it may be susceptible to thrombotic events. A thrombotic event affecting the posterior cerebral artery can affect both the cochlea and the vestibular labyrinth, accounting for the vertigo and hearing loss simultaneously experienced by this patient. This theory is further supported by evidence linking ovarian stimulation with ischemic strokes. Rizk et al. described the case of a woman who presented 11 days post embryo transfer with dense hemiplegia and hemianopia [3]. CT scan confirmed ischemic stroke. That patient also had signs of ovarian hyperstimulation syndrome. Inbar et al. described the case of a woman on clomifene citrate ovarian stimulation therapy who experienced a temporo-parietal infarct [4]. Interestingly, that patient did not show signs of ovarian hyperstimulation syndrome.

An alternative hypothesis is that the hormonal variation had a direct impact on hearing. Andreyko and Jaffe have described a case series of bilateral high-frequency hearing loss during the late luteal phase of the menstrual cycle [5], which was successfully treated with ovarian suppression. This demonstrates a link between estrogen, progesterone, and hearing. It has been speculated by Law and Moon that estrogen and progesterone alter the electrolyte balance of the inner ear and therefore may affect hearing [6]. Thus, in the case described here, hearing loss could be a direct result of the hormonal interaction with the ear, without a thrombotic trigger.

In conclusion, it is difficult to establish the exact cause of sensorineural hearing loss in this patient. On balance, a thrombotic event is more likely than an endocrine cause. It is also difficult to determine this patient's future risk should she decide to undergo further fertility treatment.

References

1. Arts HA. Differential diagnosis of sensorineural hearing loss. *Otolaryngology – Head & Neck Surgery*. St Louis, USAMO: Mosby Year Book; 1998: 2923–8.

2. Hanna GS. Sudden deafness and the contraceptive pill. *J Laryngol Otol* 1986; **100**(6): 701–6.

3. Rizk B, Meagher S, Fisher AM. Severe ovarian hyperstimulation syndrome and

cerebrovascular accidents. *Hum Reprod* 1990; **5**(6): 697–8.

4. Inbar OJ, Levran D, Mashiach S, Dor J. Ischemic stroke due to induction of ovulation with clomiphene citrate and menotropins without evidence of ovarian hyperstimulation syndrome. *Fertil Steril* 1994; **62**(5): 1075–6.

5. Andreyko JL, Jaffe RB. Use of a gonadotropin-releasing hormone agonist analogue for treatment of cyclic auditory dysfunction. *Obstet Gynecol* 1989; **74**(3 Pt 2): 506–9.

6. Law DW, Moon CE. Fluctuating hearing sensorineural hearing impairment associated with the menstrual cycle. *J Audiol Res* 1967; **7**: 373–85.

Index

Note: page numbers in *italics* refer to figures and tables.